DERMATOLOGY - LABORATORY AND CLINICAL RESEARCH

DERMATITIS

CAUSES, SYMPTOMS AND TREATMENT OPTIONS

DERMATOLOGY - LABORATORY AND CLINICAL RESEARCH

Additional books in this series can be found on Nova's website under the Series tab.

Additional e-books in this series can be found on Nova's website under the e-book tab.

DERMATOLOGY - LABORATORY AND CLINICAL RESEARCH

DERMATITIS

CAUSES, SYMPTOMS AND TREATMENT OPTIONS

CORNELIA SIGRID LISSI MÜLLER
EDITOR

NOVA BIOMEDICAL
New York

For permission to use material from this book please contact us:
Telephone 631-231-7269; Fax 631-231-8175
Web Site: http://www.novapublishers.com

Library of Congress Cataloging-in-Publication Data

ISBN: 978-1-62618-997-3

Library of Congress Control Number: 2013939113

Published by Nova Science Publishers, Inc. † New York

This work is dedicated to the memory of my mother.

Contents

Preface

Inflammatory diseases of the skin are an ever-changing field in the area of dermatology. In the selection of all chapters for this book I hope to focus on especially problematic, innovative and important areas in the field of inflammatory skin diseases. The term "dermatitis" is widely used as an umbrella for any kind of inflammation of the superficial parts of the skin, irregardless of the underlying cause. Inflammation of the skin can be of autoimmune, infectious or allergic nature and results in a distinct set of clinical symptoms, e.g. erythema, vesiculation, scaling and itching of the skin. Depending of the time course acute and chronic courses have to be divided.

In contrast to classical dermatological textbooks, chapters of this book have been selected to highlight special attributes of distinct clinical settings of cutaneous inflammation: childhood dermatitis from clinical as well as histopathological view is reviewed and excellent comprehensive information is presented on current aspects of the role of calcium in inflammatory skin diseases, the relevance of clonal T-cell populations in certain kinds of dermatitis and recent knowledge on infectious diseases as Lyme disease via clinical, diagnostic and histopathological. Last but not least chronic hand eczema and allergic contact dermatitis due to orthodontic material is discussed.

As a result of these chapters a wide-ranging summery on the increasing field of inflammation of the skin is presented and I am for sure that this book will have a prominent place in the bookshelves of clinical dermatologist.

Reading these excellent chapters of this book I learned amazing information and I am happy for the opportunity to edit this text and I am deeply grateful for the exceptional efforts of the contributing authors.

Cornelia S. L. Müller, MD

In: Dermatitis
Editor: Cornelia Sigrid Lissi Müller
ISBN: 978-1-62618-997-3

Chapter I

The Value of Skin Biopsies in the Diagnosis of Inflammatory Skin Diseases in Children

Almut Böer-Auer*
Dermatologikum Hamburg, Department of Dermatopathology,
Hamburg, Germany

Abstract

Interpretation of biopsies is integral to the diagnosis of inflammatory skin diseases, especially when the clinical appearance is not unequivocally diagnostic. Despite that, biopsies are relatively rarely taken in children. Dermatopathologists are often unfamiliar with conditions that occur only in children or that show clinical and histopathologic variations in childhood that differ from those seen in adults. The diagnostic value of skin biopsies in children with inflammatory skin diseases is summarized on the basis of a selective review of the literature. Emphasis is given to the differential diagnosis of figurate erythemas, Blaschko-linear dermatoses, exanthemas, and nodular lesions in the pediatric age group. Figurate eruptions addressed in this article include neutrophil-rich infiltrates of urticaria-like exanthemas in cryopyrin-associated periodic syndrome, eruptions in systemic juvenile idiopathic arthritis/Still's disease, atypical manifestations of Borreliosis, and the newly recognized

* Corresponding author: Phone +4940 35107578, Email boer@dermatologikum.de.

entity annular lichenoid dermatitis of youth (ALDY). Blaschko-linear dermatoses such as incontinentia pigmenti, lichen striatus, and ILVEN are presented with typical histopathology and diagnostic clues. Classic childhood exanthemas as well as generalized/systemic allergic contact dermatitis and Id-reactions are mentioned as differential diagnoses of typical exanthematic skin eruptions such as eruptive psoriasis, pityriasis rosea, or pityriasis lichenoides which also tend to appear preferentially in younger patients. Pediatric lichen planus is presented as an example of a disease with dramatic geographical/ethnic age variation; while common in India/Middle East it is hardly ever diagnosed in Europe/United States. Some examples of nodular infiltrates specific for the pediatric age group, e.g., subcutaneous fat necrosis of the newborn, subcutaneous granuloma annulare, and palmoplantar neutrophilic eccrine hidradenitis are addressed.

In conclusion, skin biopsies taken from inflammatory infiltrates in a child often help to come to a specific diagnosis and, at times, they enable early recognition of inherited systemic inflammatory syndromes or acquired autoimmune diseases. Moreover, histopathologic assessment can be the vehicle to initiate additional molecular diagnostic procedures on the same biopsy, e.g., for identification of infectious organisms. Last, thorough clinicopathological correlation helps to refine diagnostic criteria, to identify new disease entities, and to unmask flawed disease concepts in the pediatric age group.

Introduction

Histopathologic diagnosis of inflammatory skin diseases in children may be challenging for a variety of reasons: First of all, the spectrum of histologic changes is less well known given the small number of skin biopsies taken in children. Second, the clinical presentation may differ from that in seen in adults. Third, some conditions occur only in children, but most of them are rare. Fourth, the spectrum of differential diagnoses changes with the age of a patient, and last, the concepts of diseases may not be as clear due to the limited number of studies.

This chapter summarizes the results of a selective literature review on various inflammatory diseases that appear mainly in childhood and of diseases that may occur at any age but that often present differently in the pediatric population, either clinically or histopathologically. Emphasis is given to clinicopathological correlation, differential diagnoses, and to concepts of disease entities. The content of this chapter was selected based on practical importance and personal experience; it does not attempt to be all-encompassing.

Essentially, the method of histopathologic diagnosis of inflammatory skin diseases in children is the same that we use in biopsies taken from adults:

1. Categorization of the infiltrate into a basic pattern
2. Further classification according to
   (a) epidermal changes
   (b) composition of the infiltrate
   (c) deposits in the dermis
   (d) damage to the vessels etc.

Interpretation of a biopsy specimen usually should be started in "Ackerman-fashion" without looking at the clinical description and without knowing the age of the patient [1]. However, the age of the patient as well as a very basic description of clinical lesions, i.e., as figurate erythema, Blaschko-linear eruption, exanthema, or nodule is likely to change fundamentally our differential diagnostic thoughts, especially in the pediatric age group. In many cases of inflammatory infiltrates in children, clinicopathological correlation is indispensable for coming to a specific diagnosis. Therefore, the conditions are organized here according to rough clinical categories.

Figurate Erythemas

A broad variety of conditions may present as a figurate erythema in a child, among them being urticaria, lupus erythematosus, erythema annulare centrifugum, and tinea [2]. All these conditions are recognizable in sections of a biopsy specimen with identical changes in children and adults. However, the following conditions have to be included in the differential diagnoses of figurate erythemas especially when the patient is a child:

Urticaria-Like Exanthemas in Cryopyrin-Associated Periodic Syndrome

Under the heading of Cryopyrin-associated periodic syndrome, three clinical manifestations are grouped together, namely, familial cold autoinflammatory syndrome, Muckle-Wells syndrome, and CINCA syndrome

[3-7]. All of these are caused by heterozygous mutations in the NLRP3 gene. The typical clinical presentation is an urticarial exanthema that usually is not pruritic and that may remain in situ for more than 24 hours. Usually, symptoms start early in life and they are associated with fever, leukocytosis, and arthropathy, and may lead to systemic amyloidosis in adulthood. In addition, patients with Muckle-Wells syndrome develop progressive deafness. Patients with CINCA syndrome, who always have a neonatal onset, will present with CNS symptoms and with disproportionate growth and they bear a 20% risk of lethality. Early recognition of the condition is of great importance to the patients because treatment with IL-1-receptor antibodies is now available. It improves the condition dramatically and also helps to prevent the sequelae of systemic amyloidosis [3].

Histopathologic changes demonstrate the pattern designated as "neutrophil-rich urticaria" which is typified by a perivascular infiltrate of lymphocytes and neutrophils accompanied by neutrophils in the interstitial dermis (Figure 1A and B). While there can be slight nuclear dust of neutrophils, signs of vasculitis such as fibrin deposition in the vessel wall, are absent.

Eruption in Systemic Juvenile Idiopathic Arthritis/Still's Disease

Systemic juvenile idiopathic arthritis or Still's disease is classified as a subset of juvenile idiopathic arthritis. It is defined by the presence of arthritis in one or more joints associated with spiking fever (typically daily with spike in the evening) persisting for at least 15 days together with one or more of the following manifestations: exanthema, generalized lymphadenopathy, hepatomegaly, and/or splenomegaly, or serositis. The course of the disease can be highly variable, monocyclic, polycyclic with relapses followed by intervals of remission, or unremitting. In about half of the patients chronic destructive arthritis may develop [8-9]. Laboratory tests show leukocytosis with neutrophilia, thrombocytosis, high C-reactive protein and erythrocyte sedimentation rate. A nonpruritic, transient, erythematous, urticaria-like eruption occurs in many patients together with arthralgia, fever, and leukocytosis [8-9]. Red dermographism is typical of the condition. Sometimes, the skin eruption precedes the arthralgia for months or years.

Microscopically, the changes are similar to those seen in urticarial eruptions of Cryopyrin-associated periodic syndrome showing also the pattern of a "neutrophil-rich urticaria". In addition, neutrophils may be found in eccrine ductal epithelium (Figure 1C and D) [10].

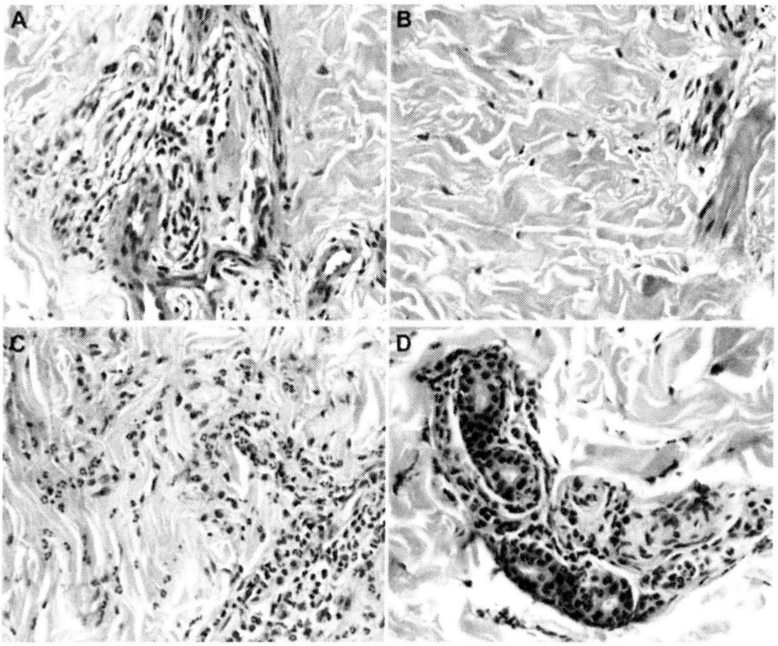

Figure 1. The pattern of "neutrophil rich urticaria" is typified by perivascular infiltrates of lymphocytes and neutrophils combined with interstitial lymphocytes, eosinophils are lacking. A and B. Cryopyrin-associated periodic syndrome: Some nuclear dust of neutrophils is present, but no fibrin is seen in the walls of vessels. C and D. Systemic juvenile idiopathic arthritis (Still's disease): Neutrophils may be present in the walls of eccrine ducts.

Borreliosis

Borreliosis is the most common acquired tick-borne infection in Europe in both, children and adults. However, the clinical presentation in children is often atypical, e.g., patchy facial erythema which may be bilateral, disseminated patchy erythema, or multiple erythemata migrantia [11-14]. These manifestations are a reflection of early hematogenous spread of the organism which is often accompanied by malaise and even by neurological symptoms. Early in the course of Borreliosis, the serology is often negative or not unequivocally diagnostic so that the diagnosis is based either on clinical inspection alone or on clinicopathological correlation.

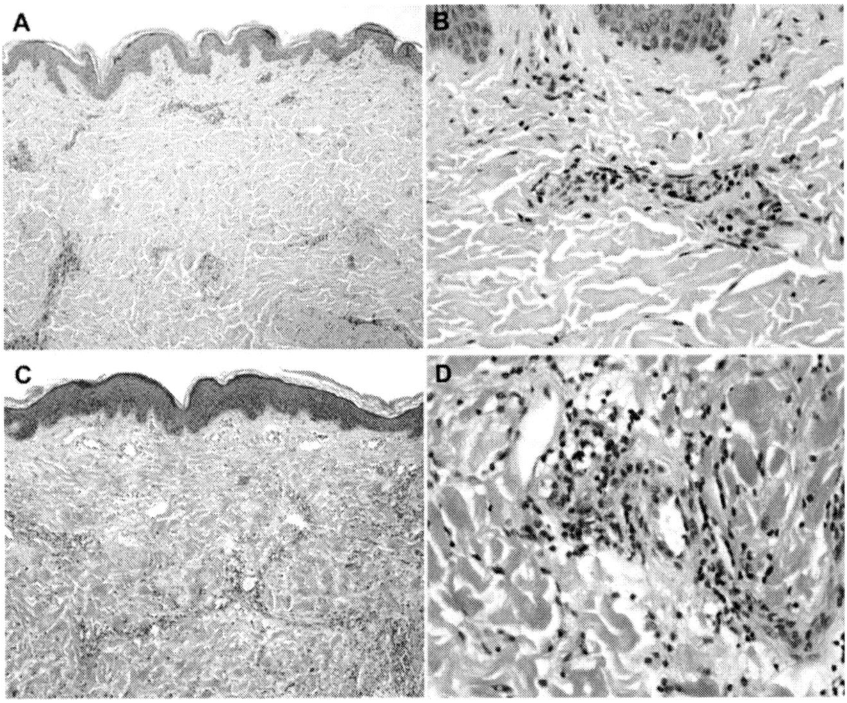

Figure 2. Plasma cell-poor infiltrates in two children with PCR-proven Borreliosis. A and B. Erythema migrans: Sparse infiltrate of lymphocytes. C and D. Acrodermatitis chronica atrophicans: Perivascular and interstitial infiltrates of lymphocytes together with marked thickening of collagen bundles.

Histopathologically, a broad variation of changes can be seen in Borreliosis of the skin. In early lesions the infiltrate may be very sparse and consists of lymphocytes only (Figure 2A and B). Perivascular and interstitial and infiltrates are usually deep, reaching the subcutis, even when they are sparse. In denser infiltrates, the phenotype may be T- or B-cell dominated, plasma cell counts range from absent to prominent, and sometimes interstitial histiocytes are numerous [15]. In late lesions of cutaneous Borreliosis, so-called acrodermatitis chronica atrophicans, thickened collagen bundles are a prominent finding (Figure 2C and D).

If clinicopathological correlation and serology is inconclusive, PCR for Borrelia-specific DNA can be performed on paraffin-embedded biopsies to confirm the diagnosis of Borreliosis [16]. In any case of "deep figurate erythema"/ "deep gyrate erythema"/"erythema annulare centrifugum-deep type" in a child, Borreliosis should be excluded by Serology and/or PCR.

Erythrokeratodermia Variabilis

Erythrokeratodermia variabilis is an inherited disorder characterized by erythematous macules and plaques, stationary or migratory, associated with nonmigratory hyperkeratoses. It usually is present at birth or occurs during the first year but it may occasionally begin later in childhood or even in early adulthood. Lesions preferentially affect the face, buttocks, and extensor surfaces of the limbs. Palmoplantar keratoderma occurs in about half the cases, but hair, nails, and teeth are not affected [17]. The cause of the disease has been identified as a mutation in the connexin genes GJB3/GJB4 on Chromosome 1p35 [18-20]. This genetic defect has linked erythrokeratodermia variabilis to progressive symmetric erythrokeratodermia and Greither disease, also known as keratosis palmoplantaris transgrediens et progrediens.

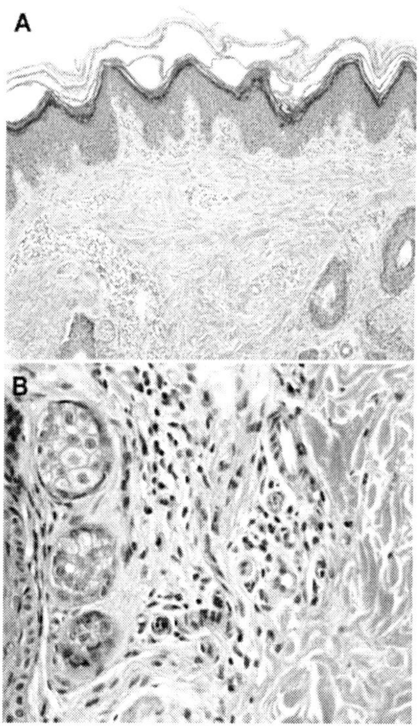

Figure 3A and B. Infiltrate in a child with erythrokeratodermia variabilis: Perivascular and periadnexal infiltrates of lymphocytes and histiocytes with few mast cells together with papillomatosis and hyperkeratosis of the epidermis.

Histologically, figurate erythema of erythrokeratodermia variabilis is typified by perivascular and periadnexal infiltrates of lymphocytes and histiocytes with few mast cells (Figure 3). A clue to the diagnosis is papillomatosis and hyperkeratosis of the epidermis which may be misinterpreted as features of lichen simplex or as site specific change when the biopsy is taken from an area close to a joint.

Annular Lichenoid Dermatitis of Youth (ALDY)

Annular lichenoid dermatitis of youth is a relatively recently described disease of unknown cause and pathogenesis [21-27]. Patients present themselves with asymptomatic erythematous macules and annular patches with a red-brownish border and central hypopigmentation. Typical sites are the groin and flanks. While the disease was described first in adolescents and young adults, it has now been observed also in older adults [22]. No T-cell clonality was identified in any of the cases and Borrelia serology was negative. Patch tests gave no positive results [21-27].

The histopathologic findings of this condition seem to be highly distinctive with an irregular acanthosis combined with a lichenoid lymphocytic dermatitis with numerous necrotic keratinocytes [21-22].

Annular Erythema of Infancy

Review of the literature in regard to the term "annular erythema of infancy" reveals a heterogeneous group of infiltrates. Lymphocytic, eosinophil-rich, and neutrophilic infiltrates have been described under the same heading suggesting that more than one entity is found under that designation [28-33]. It is likely that, apart from patients with neonatal lupus, also some with CAPS or with Borreliosis were previously labeled with the diagnosis of annular erythema of infancy.

Blaschko-Linear Dermatoses

Blaschko lines reflect the paths of cell migration and clonal expansion during embryologic and fetal development [2, 34-35]. Numerous conditions may present themselves in Blaschko-linear distribution such as epidermal nevi, nevus sebaceous, hypomelanosis of Ito, but also inflammatory infiltrates. In childhood, the following conditions are of special importance (Figure 4):

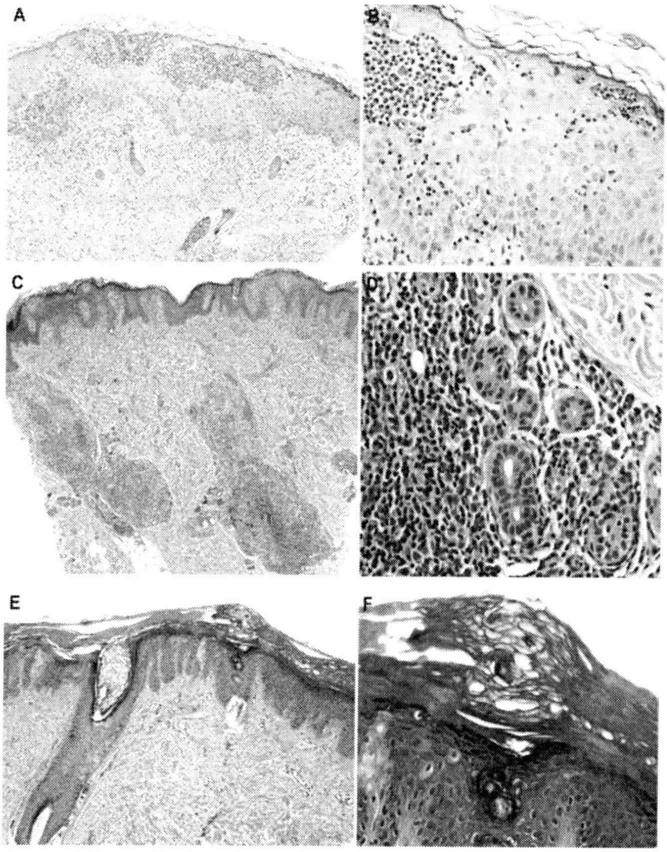

Figure 4. Diagnostic patterns in Blaschko-linear dermatoses. A and B. Incontinentia pigmenti, early stage: Intraepidermal vesicles filled with eosinophils together with dyskeratotic cells. C and D. Lichen striatus: Interface dermatitis with eccrocentric infiltrates. E and F. ILVEN: Sharp demarcation between orthokeratosis and parakeratosis, orthokeratosis above acrosyringia/infundibula, and a dermal infiltrate.

Incontinentia Pigmenti

Incontinentia pigmenti is a genodermatosis inherited in X-chromosomal-dominant fashion. The mutation has been located to the NEMO gene (Xq28, NF-kappa B) [36]. The condition affects only girls, except rare mosaicism or Klinefelter syndrome and it manifests itself already shortly after birth [37]. The clinical features pass through typical stages with erythematous vesicles (1.-4. months), hyperkeratotic plaques (2.-6. months), hyperpigmentation

(7.months-12 years), and hypopigmented atrophic lines (6 years-adults) [38]. Exacerbation can be seen during infections [39-40]. In approximately 80% of all patients the genodermatosis also affects other organs such as the eyes, teeth, CNS, skeleton, and heart [41-42]. The prognosis chiefly depends on the degree of CNS involvement.

The histopathologic findings of incontinentia pigmenti vary according to the stage in the process: At the beginning, spongiotic vesicles are joined by intraepidermal eosinophils and dyskeratotic cells combined with a superficial perivascular infiltrate dominated by eosinophils (Figure 4A and B). Later, hyperkeratosis, hyperplasia, and papillomatosis develop and dyskeratotic cells of various numbers can be found at all levels of the epidermis. At a late stage, melanophages are present in the papillary dermis. Even in adulthood, necrotic keratinocytes in the epidermis or dermis are a clue to the diagnosis of incontinentia pigmenti but at that stage, melanocytes are reduced in number, some fibrosis is found in the dermis and hair follicles are atrophic [43].

Lichen Striatus

Lichen striatus is a well-defined clinicopathological entity in children, but it is not a disease restricted to childhood [43-49]. The clinical presentation is that of a papular or papulovesicular eruption that presents itself along the lines of Blaschko. While it typically presents as one line on an extremity, it may also be multilinear and it may involve more than one limb, trunk, and the face. Occasionally and more commonly in adults than in children, lesions are pruritic. Hypopigmented and hyperpigmented variants occur especially in darker skin types. Typically the eruption resolves within months or years but it may relapse, a feature described more commonly in adults than in children. Occasionally, familial cases have been reported.

The histopathological key features of lichen striatus is a lichenoid interface dermatitis with eccrocentric infiltrates (Figure 4C and D) [49]. The accompanying epidermal changes show broad variation in regard to degree of spongiosis, and the number of necrotics. The subepidermal infiltrate may be dense and lichenoid or sparse. In some cases, spongiosis is so prominent that necrotic keratinocytes are less obvious [44, 46, 49]. The perieccrine infiltrates are sometimes accompanied by eccrine glandular hyperplasia similar to that seen in some cases of syringotropic mycosis fungoides.

Pediatric Blaschkitis

Relatively recently, a new entity termed "Pediatric Blaschkitis" was postulated based on two patients reported in the literature [50-51]. In this context it is important to know that the condition "Blaschkitis" of adulthood was suggested by Grosshans in 1990 based on just one single patient [52]. His reasons for separating "Blaschkitis" from lichen striatius were occurrence in adulthood, location on the trunk, multilinearity, pruritus, rapid resolution and relapse, and histopathologic changes of prominent spongiosis and vesiculation. Grosshans admitted that necrotic keratinocytes were rare but not absent in this setting. In the meantime, studies have shown that lichen striatus may be papulovesicular, pruritic, multilinear, recurrent, and devoid of necrosis with prominent spongiosis and that it presents in both, children and adults [44, 46, 49]. Therefore, the criteria for differentiation of lichen striatus from another quite similar condition termed "Blaschkitis" are not compelling, neither in adults nor in chidren [48, 53].

Inflammatory Linear Verrucous Epidermal Nevus (ILVEN)

ILVEN is an epidermal nevus that usually appears in the 1st -5th year of life [54]. It has a chronic course with episodic exacerbation of inflammation. Clinically, the condition presents with pruritic psoriasiform papules and plaques in Blaschko-linear distribution. It has long been an issue of controversy whether ILVEN represents a linear manifestation of psoriasis but more recently immunohistochemical and ultrastructural studies as well as analysis of epidermal proteins have demonstrated differences between lesions ILVEN and lesions of psoriasis [55-61]. Histopathologically, psoriasiform acanthosis, sharp demarcation between stubby zones of orthokeratosis and parakeratosis and orthokeratosis above acrosyringia/infundibula are typical of ILVEN (Figure 4E and F). The accompanying dermal infiltrate is quite variable. Of course, the main differential diagnosis of ILVEN is psoriasis which may present itself also in Blaschko-linear arrangement or it may manifest itself in a preexisting epidermal nevus by way of Köbnerization. In both settings, the histopathology is that of psoriasis, in the latter case together with more pronounced papillation. Both conditions are very different form ILVEN, which is a true epidermal nevus with specific histological features. However, some cases published in the literature under the diagnosis of ILVEN seem to represent, in fact, Blaschko-linear manifestations of psoriasis [62].

Exanthemas

The differential diagnoses of exanthemas in children include classical childhood exanthemas such as measles or scarlet fever, but also inflammatory skin conditions like psoriasis, pityriasis rosea and pityriasis lichenoides which may occur triggered by a preceding infection. For the most part, histopathologic changes in children and adults affected by these conditions are the same. Interestingly, ethnic differences are encountered in the incidence of some exanthematic eruptions, e.g., lichen planus of childhood in the Indian and Middle Eastern population. Moreover, contact allergies in children are increasing and may present as a generalized eruption. Id-reactions such as papular urticaria as a response to insect bites are also common in childhood.

Viral Exanthemas

Classical exanthemas of childhood include the eruptions seen in measles (rubeola), scarlet fever, rubella, erythema infectiosum (fifth's disease), and roseola [63]. However, all of these conditions present themselves usually in such typical fashion that they are rarely biopsied. Many other viral infections, e.g. those caused by coxsackieviruses, echoviruses, and enteroviruses may also be accompanied by exanthems. These eruptions are usually self- limiting and resolve spontaneously within a week. Common associations are fever and lymphadenopathy.

Histopathologic features in biopsies taken from these eruptions are usually not specific. The most common feature is a sparse perivascular dermatitis made up of lymphocytes. Sometimes, additional changes are suggestive of a specific infection [1]. For example, multinucleated epithelial cells in the absence of ballooning or steel gray nuclei may be seen in measles, focal spongiosis can be seen in Gianotti-Crosti syndrome, and spongiosis joined by ballooning and necrosis (but devoid of acantholysis) is suggestive of hand-foot-and-mouth disease. [1]

Lichen Planus

Lichen planus is a common inflammatory disease of the skin of adults, whereas it is rare in children [64-76]. However, there are ethnic differences in the incidence of lichen planus in childhood. The vast majority of larger studies on childhood lichen planus come from India [66-67, 75]. It has been suggested that the increased incidence is the result of an interplay of ethnic, genetic, and climatic factors. Only few studies on childhood lichen planus were undertaken outside India [71, 74]. From Germany and the United States, lichen planus in children was reported exclusively in the form of case reports [64].

The typical age of children with lichen planus is between 5 and 9 years while the disease is extremely uncommon in infants. Just as in the adult population, the lower extremities are often the sites of onset of the disease [67]. The majority of children presents with classic exanthematic distribution of lesions [66-67, 75]. Hypertrophic and linear forms of the disease constitute a minority of cases [66-67, 75]. Mostly spared are palms, soles, nails, scalp, and mucosa. Genitalia and face may be involved at times and hyperpigmentation common, presumably because of the ethnic skin type of affected patients [66-67].

In regard to the etiology of lichen planus in children, an association with vaccination has been described in several reports [69, 74, 76]. Some children developed lichen planus after simultaneous measles-mumps-rubella and diphtheria-tetanus-pertussis-polio vaccinations [76]. Others possibly reacted to anti-hepatitis B vaccination [69, 74]. One child developed lichen planus after receiving growth hormone for dwarfism [73]. There is no universally accepted treatment for lichen planus in childhood. Patients in the literature were said to have responded favorably to topical corticosteroids, systemic flucortolon, or systemic dapsone [64, 72]. A few patients of Arab descent were also treated with UVB phototherapy with good results [72]. Acitretin in the dose of 0.5mg/kg/day for a few weeks showed marked improvement in few patients reported by Merigou D et al. and Brockow et al.[65, 70].

Histopathologic findings of lichen planus in adults and children are those of lichenoid interface dermatitis with variable numbers of necrotic keratinocytes in the basal layer, jagged appearance of the rete ridges, wedge-shaped hypergranulosis and compact orthokeratosis. The dermal infiltrate is monopolized by lymphocytes. Comparison of histopathologic findings in adults and children revealed a number of subtle differences, among them an increased number of necrotic keratinocytes, denser and deeper infiltrates, more adnexocentrism, and a few neutrophils, eosinophils, or plasma cells admixed in the infiltrate (Figure 5). These slight differences seem to suggest that lichen planus in children is pathogenetically different from lichen planus of adults [64].

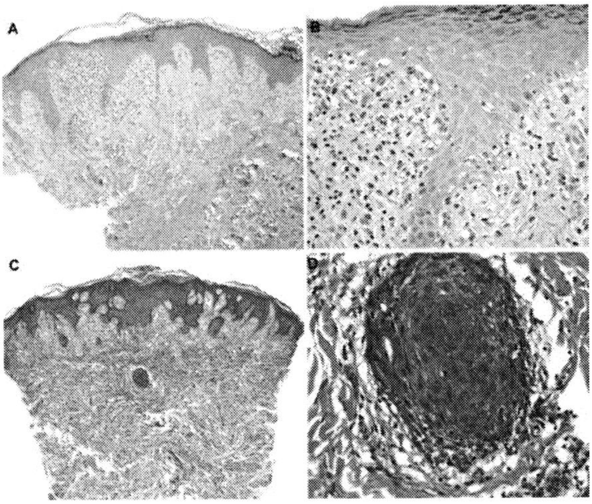

Figure 5. Lichen planus in children from the Middle East and India. A and B. The infiltrate is dominated by lymphocytes but also houses a few neutrophils. C and D. The infiltrate is extending into the mid dermis and it is adnexocentric.

Generalized/Systemic Allergic Contact Dermatitis, Id-Reaction

Allergic contact dermatitis is an acquired skin disease mediated by a type IV immune mechanism. Patch testing is the diagnostic standard procedure for the identification of sensitizing allergens. The overall incidence rate of positive patch test results in children is increasing [77-80]. It is thought that the increased rates may be due to increases in utilization of personal health products in everyday life that contain certain allergens and to the fact that children are becoming exposed to a wider variety of allergens at a younger age. Allergic contact dermatitis in childhood may have important implications for the patient as it may affect decisions regarding future occupation in adulthood [77]. Early diagnosis of contact allergy by way of patch test is associated with an improved quality of life and increased response to treatment [77, 81]. If an allergen is identified, simple avoidance is the most effective treatment modality. In any case of "refractory atopic dermatitis" in a child, allergic contact dermatitis should be considered as a possible diagnosis. Nickel is the most common allergen among children and adolescents. Clinical presentation may be localized, generalized or even systemic [82-83].

Histopathologically, the changes of allergic contact dermatitis in pediatric patients are no different from those seen in adults. Depending on the duration of the disease, spongiotic or spongiotic-psoriasiform dermatitis with a superficial infiltrate of lymphocytes is typical [1]. Eosinophils in the infiltrate can be a clue to the diagnosis but absence of eosinophils does not rule out the possibility of a contact allergen as the causative agent of an eruption. Because the condition is usually itchy, changes of lichen simplex chronicus may be superimposed on the spongiotic dermatitis [1]. In systemic manifestations of contact allergies, the presentation in the skin may be that of an Id-reaction typified by a wedge-shaped superficial and deep infiltrate with focal spongiosis similar to what can be seen in insect bite reactions [1, 83].

Id-reactions to other stimuli such as dermatophyte infections, infestations, or arthropod assaults are histologically largely indistinguishable from the findings seen in systemic manifestations of contact allergies (Figure 6).[1, 84-85]. Generalized hypersensitivity to bites from certain insects such as mosquitoes, gnats, fleas, mites, and bedbugs are also known under the designation papular urticaria [85-86]. Papular urticaria is common in childhood and presents with symmetrically distributed pruritic papules and papulovesicles that may occur more than one week after the sting of an insect.

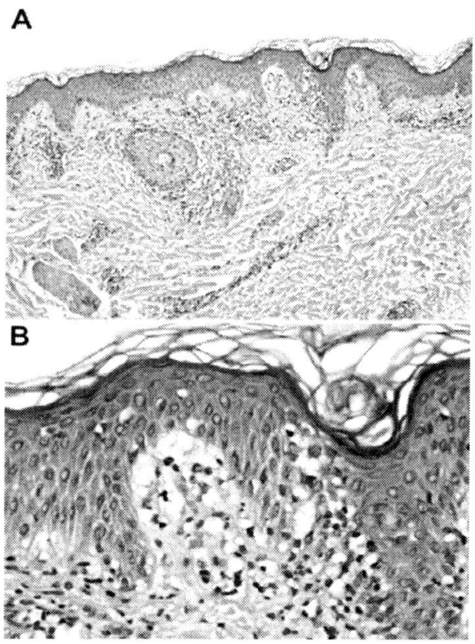

Figure 6. Id-reaction occurring in a boy one week after an insect bite. The changes are very similar to those seen in a bite: A wedge-shaped perivascular and perifollicular infiltrate of lymphocytes and histiocytes is accompanied by focal spongiosis. Few eosinophils are present in the infiltrate.

Nodules

Nodular skin lesions in children most commonly are identified as cysts, neoplasms, or hamartomas on histopathological examination. Apart from that, some inflammatory conditions also may present clinically with indurated nodules in a child:

Idiopathic Palmoplantar Hidradenitis

Idiopathic palmoplantar eccrine hidradenitis is characterized by painful erythematous nodules of abrupt onset on the soles and, less commonly, on the palms of young children [87-90]. Lesions typically occur after intense physical activity sometimes combined with exposure to cold.

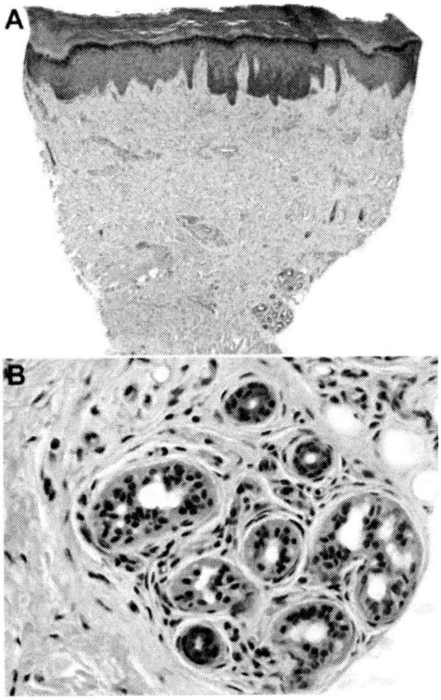

Figure 7. Idiopathic palmoplantar hidradenitis, late stage. A sparse infiltrate of lymphocytes is present in and around eccrine glands. Few necrotic epithelial cells can be identified within the gland.

The course is usually self-limiting with avoidance of triggering factors but sometimes there is more than one episode. Histopathologically, the changes are similar to that seen in eccrine neutrophilic hidradenitis as it presents in adult patients as a response to some chemotherapeutic agents. A dense infiltrate of neutrophils is seen in and around eccrine glands [90]. Some necrotic cells can be identified within the eccrine glands. If, however, a biopsy is taken late in the course, a sparse infiltrate of lymphocytes in and around eccrine glands, sometimes still associated with a few necrotic epithelial cells is seen (Figure 7).

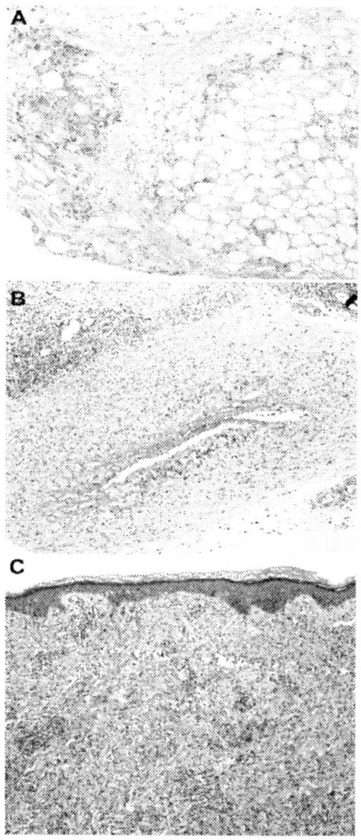

Figure 8. Important patterns of nodular granulomatous infiltrates in children: A: Subcutaneous fat necrosis of the newborn. Needle-shaped clefts in radial arrangement in histiocytes scattered throughout subcutaneous lobules, together with a granulomatous infiltrate with multinucleate and foamy histiocytes. B: Subcutaneous granuloma annulare. Palisaded granulomas around large areas of basophilic degeneration of collagen in the subcutis together with increased amounts of connective tissue mucin and nuclear dust of neutrophils between degenerated collagen bundles. C: Sarcoidal granulomas in a child with PCR-proven Leishmaniasis caused by *L. infantum*.

Subcutaneous Fat Necrosis

Subcutaneous fat necrosis of the newborn is a relatively uncommon self limited condition caused by perinatal hypoxemia, hypothermia, or local hypoperfusion [91-93]. Affected newborns present with nodules and plaques on trunk, arms, buttocks, thighs, and cheeks. Sometimes, hypercalcemia may be accompanying and may require treatment and follow up of a patient.

Histopathologically, needle-shaped clefts in radial arrangement in histiocytes scattered throughout subcutaneous lobules, but also sometimes in adipocytes are typical of the condition (Figure 8A). A granulomatous infiltrate with multinucleate and foamy histiocytes is accompanying [1, 94].

Subcutaneous Granuloma Annulare

Granuloma annulare is a common disease in children as well as in adults, but the subcutaneous nodular variant is much more common in childhood [95-98]. The clinical presentation is that of a solitary nodule or few nodules on the anterior aspects of the lower extremities, hands, head, and buttocks of young children. In some cases, an association with diabetes mellitus has been documented [95]. Lesions usually regress spontaneously, but occasionally there is recurrence.

In conventional lesions of granuloma annulare the infiltrate is located in the superficial dermis and shows palisaded or interstitial infiltrates of histiocytes accompanied by perivascular infiltrates of lymphocytes sometimes joined by eosinophils. Usually, mucin can be identified in the center of palisaded granulomas. In contrast, subcutaneous lesions of granuloma annulare show palisaded granulomas around large areas of basophilic degeneration of collagen in the subcutis (Figure 8B) [97-98]. In addition, increased amounts of connective tissue mucin and nuclear dust of neutrophils is present between degenerated collagen bundles. In only 25% of the patients, lesions of subcutaneous granuloma annulare coexist with classic findings of granuloma annulare in the dermis.

Cutaneous Leishmaniasis

Leishmaniasis is a protozoan diseases caused by Leishmania species which are transmitted by the bite of certain species of the sand fly [99-101].

Clinically leishmaniasis shows a broad spectrum of clinical manifestations including localized cutaneous lesions, mucocutaneous involvement, or disseminated and potentially lethal infections. The parasites are mainly found in South Asia, the Horn of Africa, Central and South America and in the Mediterranean region. In non-endemic countries leishmaniasis is a disease of travelers and migrants. While some species of leishmania tend to involve only the skin (e.g., L. tropica), others bare the risk of mucocutaneous or systemic infection (e.g., L. infantum). Outdoor activities in endemic regions put unaware individuals, especially children, at risk of being bitten and infected. For infection with L. infantum it has been shown that children below the age of 3 years have a higher risk to develop visceral disease compared with older children and adults, a finding that has been attributed to age related differences in T-cell immunity [100]. Therefore it is important to consider a diagnosis of leishmaniasis in any child that presents with a single or few nodules especially when lesions are located on uncovered skin areas and when there is a history of travels or residence in endemic areas [99].

Classic histopathological findings of cutaneous leishmaniasis are those of a tuberculoid granulomatous dermatitis with plasma cells and evidence of amastigotes in histiocytes or free in the tissue [1]. Lesions are often ulcerated and crusted. However, it has been demonstrated that cutaneous leishmaniasis may also present with other types of granulomas including sarcoidal, palisaded, interstitial, and foreign body types (Figure 8C) [99, 102]. In such cases, the load of organisms is often low and a specific diagnosis can only be reached with additional culture or with PCR. More recently, PCR for leishmania specific DNA has also become very reliable when performed on paraffin embedded tissue. Even specific subtypes can be identified in such specimens so that culture may not be necessary. Exact typing should be performed because it helps to identify patients at risk for mucocutaneous and systemic infections and it is also important to select the most appropriate treatment [103].

Conclusion

The literature summarized in this chapter provides compelling evidence, that skin biopsies are a helpful tool in the diagnosis of dermatitides in childhood. Even though dermatologists are often reluctant to biopsy children, the trauma of a skin biopsy has to be weighed against the potential harm of a delayed diagnosis. Skin biopsies may provide important clues to the diagnosis of inherited systemic inflammatory syndromes and to acquired autoimmune diseases in which early diagnosis can prevent severe and lifelong sequelae. In the setting of infectious diseases, Borreliosis and leishmaniasis are excellent examples for the broad variation of morphological changes clinically and histopathologically, which may be caused, in part, by age related differences in the immune response. In such cases, the patterns of infiltrates observed in a biopsy specimen can be the springboard to initiate additional molecular investigations which permit a specific diagnosis, e.g., identification of organism-specific DNA by way of PCR techniques. Thorough clinico-pathological correlation remains a very important diagnostic procedure in the pediatric age group, especially for conditions of unknown etiology and pathogenesis. It is essential for the selection of the most effective treatment, it helps to identify new disease entities, and it provides the basis to unmask flawed disease concepts.

References

[1] Ackerman, AB; Böer, A; Benin, B; Gottlieb, GJ. Histologic Diagnosis of Inflammatory Skin Diseases. An Algorithmic Method Based on Pattern Analysis 3rd Editition. ed. New York City: Ardor Scribendi, Ltd., 2005, ISBN 1-893357-25-2.

[2] Höger, PH. Kinderdermatologie. 2nd. Edition ed. Stuttgart: Schattauer, 2007.

[3] Kone-Paut, I; Piram, M. Targeting interleukin-1beta in CAPS (cryopyrin-associated periodic) syndromes: what did we learn? *Autoimmun Rev.*, 2012, Nov;12(1), 77-80.

[4] Krause, K; Grattan, CE; Bindslev-Jensen, C; Gattorno, M; Kallinich, T; de Koning, HD; et al. How not to miss autoinflammatory diseases masquerading as urticaria. *Allergy.*, 2012, Dec, 67(12), 1465-74.

[5] Ombrello, MJ; Remmers, EF; Sun, G; Freeman, AF; Datta, S; Torabi-Parizi, P; et al. Cold urticaria, immunodeficiency, and autoimmunity related to PLCG2 deletions. *N Engl J Med.*, 2012 Jan 26, 366(4), 330-8.

[6] Posch, C; Kaulfersch, W; Rappersberger, K. Cryopyrin-Associated Periodic Syndrome. *Pediatr Dermatol.*, 2012, Aug 14.

[7] Wanderer, AA. Exanthem with cryopyrin associated periodic syndromes and consideration of IL-1 targeted therapy for neutrophilic predominant urticaria. *Allergol Int.*, 2010 Sep, 59(3), 321, author reply -2.

[8] Frosch, M; Roth, J. New insights in systemic juvenile idiopathic arthritis--from pathophysiology to treatment. *Rheumatology* (Oxford)., 2008, Feb, 47(2), 121-5.

[9] Mellins, ED; Macaubas, C; Grom, AA. Pathogenesis of systemic juvenile idiopathic arthritis: some answers, more questions. *Nat Rev Rheumatol.*, 2011, Jul, 7(7), 416-26.

[10] Frosch, M; Metze, D; Foell, D; Vogl, T; Sorg, C; Sunderkotter, C; et al. Early activation of cutaneous vessels and epithelial cells is characteristic of acute systemic onset juvenile idiopathic arthritis. *Exp Dermatol.*, 2005, Apr, 14(4), 259-65.

[11] Andres, C; Ziai, M; Bruckbauer, H; Ring, J; Hofmann, H. Acrodermatitis chronica atrophicans in two children. *Int J Dermatol.*, 2010, Feb, 49(2), 180-3.

[12] Hofmann, H. [The variable spectrum of cutaneous Lyme borreliosis. Diagnosis and therapy]. *Hautarzt.*, 2012, May, 63(5), 381-9.

[13] Huppertz, HI. Childhood Lyme borreliosis in Europe. *Eur J Pediatr.*, 1990, Sep,149(12), 814-21.

[14] Krischer, S; Ott, H; Barker, M; Frank, J; Erdmann, S. [Multilocular erythema migrans in borreliosis]. *Klin Padiatr.*, 2004 Jul-Aug, 216(4), 236-7.

[15] Moreno, C; Kutzner, H; Palmedo, G; Goerttler, E; Carrasco, L; Requena, L. Interstitial granulomatous dermatitis with histiocytic pseudorosettes: a new histopathologic pattern in cutaneous borreliosis. Detection of Borrelia burgdorferi DNA sequences by a highly sensitive PCR-ELISA. *J Am Acad Dermatol.*, 2003, Mar, 48(3), 376-84.

[16] Boer, A; Bresch, M; Dayrit, J; Falk, TM. Erythema migrans: a reassessment of diagnostic criteria for early cutaneous manifestations of borreliosis with particular emphasis on clonality investigations. *Br J Dermatol.*, 2007, Jun, 156(6), 1263-71.

[17] Ishida-Yamamoto, A; McGrath, JA; Lam, H; Iizuka, H; Friedman, RA; Christiano, AM. The molecular pathology of progressive symmetric erythrokeratoderma: a frameshift mutation in the loricrin gene and perturbations in the cornified cell envelope. Am *J Hum Genet.*, 1997, Sep, 61(3), 581-9.

[18] Richard, G; Brown, N; Rouan, F; Van der Schroeff, JG; Bijlsma, E; Eichenfield, LF; et al. Genetic heterogeneity in erythrokeratodermia variabilis: novel mutations in the connexin gene GJB4 (Cx30.3) and genotype-phenotype correlations. *J Invest Dermatol.*, 2003, Apr, 120(4), 601-9.

[19] Richard, G; Brown, N; Smith, LE; Terrinoni, A; Melino, G; Mackie, RM; et al. The spectrum of mutations in erythrokeratodermias--novel and de novo mutations in GJB3. *Hum Genet.*, 2000, Mar,106(3), 321-9.

[20] van Steensel, MA; Oranje, AP; van der Schroeff, JG; Wagner, A; van Geel, M. The missense mutation G12D in connexin30.3 can cause both erythrokeratodermia variabilis of Mendes da Costa and progressive symmetric erythrokeratodermia of Gottron. *Am J Med Genet A.*, 2009, Feb 15, 149A(4), 657-61.

[21] Annessi, G; Paradisi, M; Angelo, C; Perez, M; Puddu, P; Girolomoni, G. Annular lichenoid dermatitis of youth. *J Am Acad Dermatol.*, 2003, Dec, 49(6), 1029-36.

[22] Cesinaro, AM; Sighinolfi, P; Greco, A; Garagnani, L; Conti, A; Fantini, F. Annular lichenoid dermatitis of youth ... and beyond: a series of 6 cases. *Am J Dermatopathol.*, 2009, May, 31(3), 263-7.

[23] de la Torre, C; Florez, A; Fernandez-Redondo, V. Negative results of patch testing with standard and textile series in a case of annular lichenoid dermatitis of youth. *J Am Acad Dermatol.*, 2005, Jul, 53(1), 172-3.

[24] Durdu, M; Akyilmaz, M; Tuncer, I. Annular lichenoid dermatitis of youth. *Pediatr Dermatol.*, 2007, Sep-Oct, 24(5), 582-4.

[25] Huh, W; Kanitakis, J. Annular lichenoid dermatosis of youth: report of the first Japanese case and published work review. J Dermatol., 2010, Jun, 37(6), 531-3.

[26] Kleikamp, S; Kutzner, H; Frosch, PJ. Annular lichenoid dermatitis of youth--a further case in a 12-year-old girl. *J Dtsch Dermatol Ges.*, 2008, Aug, 6(8), 653-6.

[27] Sans, V; Leaute-Labreze, C; Vergier, B; Taieb, A. A further case of annular lichenoid dermatitis of youth: role of the anti-hepatitis B immunization? *Pediatr Dermatol.*, 2008, Sep-Oct, 25(5), 577-9.

[28] Annessi, G; Signoretti, S; Angelo, C; Paradisi, M; Puddu, P. Neutrophilic figurate erythema of infancy. *Am J Dermatopathol.*, 1997, Aug, 19(4), 403-6.

[29] Hebert, AA; Esterly, NB. Annular erythema of infancy. *J Am Acad Dermatol.*, 1986, Feb, 14(2 Pt 2), 339-43.

[30] Kunz, M; Hamm, K; Brocker, EB; Hamm, H. [Annular erythema in childhood--a new eosinophilic dermatosis]. *Hautarzt.*, 1998, Feb, 49(2), 131-4.

[31] Patrizi, A; Savoia, F; Varotti, E; Gaspari, V; Passarini, B; Neri, I. Neutrophilic figurate erythema of infancy. *Pediatr Dermatol.*, 2008, Mar-Apr, 25(2), 255-60.
[32] Stachowitz, S; Abeck, D; Schmidt, T; Ring, J. Persistent annular erythema of infancy associated with intestinal Candida colonization. *Clin Exp Dermatol.*, 2000, Jul, 25(5), 404-5.
[33] Wong, LC; Kakakios, A; Rogers, M. Congenital annular erythema persisting in a 15-year-old girl. *Australas J Dermatol.*, 2002, Feb, 43(1), 55-61.
[34] Moss, C. Mosaicism and linear lesions. al. BJe, editor: *Mosby eds.*; 2003.
[35] Blaschko, A. Die Nervenverteilung in der Haut in ihre Beziehung zu den Erkrankungen der Haut. Beilage zu den Verhandlungen der Deutschen Dermatologischen Gesellschaft VII Congress, Breslau 1901.
[36] Aradhya, S; Woffendin, H; Jakins, T; Bardaro, T; Esposito, T; Smahi, A; et al. A recurrent deletion in the ubiquitously expressed NEMO (IKK-gamma) gene accounts for the vast majority of incontinentia pigmenti mutations. *Hum Mol Genet.*, 2001, Sep 15, 10(19), 2171-9.
[37] Garcia-Dorado, J; de Unamuno, P; Fernandez-Lopez, E; Salazar Veloz, J; Armijo, M. Incontinentia pigmenti: XXY male with a family history. *Clin Genet.*, 1990, Aug, 38(2), 128-38.
[38] Hadj-Rabia, S; Rimella, A; Smahi, A; Fraitag, S; Hamel-Teillac, D; Bonnefont, JP; et al. Clinical and histologic features of incontinentia pigmenti in adults with nuclear factor-kappaB essential modulator gene mutations. *J Am Acad Dermatol.*, 2011, Mar, 64(3), 508-15.
[39] Alikhan, A; Lee, AD; Swing, D; Carroll, C; Yosipovitch, G. Vaccination as a probable cause of incontinentia pigmenti reactivation. *Pediatr Dermatol.*, 2010, Jan-Feb, 27(1), 62-4.
[40] Bodak, N; Hadj-Rabia, S; Hamel-Teillac, D; de Prost, Y; Bodemer, C. Late recurrence of inflammatory first-stage lesions in incontinentia pigmenti: an unusual phenomenon and a fascinating pathologic mechanism. *Arch Dermatol.*, 2003, Feb, 139(2), 201-4.
[41] Meuwissen, ME; Mancini, GM. Neurological findings in incontinentia pigmenti; a review. *Eur J Med Genet.*, 2012, May, 55(5), 323-31.
[42] O'Doherty, M; Mc Creery, K; Green, AJ; Tuwir, I; Brosnahan, D. Incontinentia pigmenti--ophthalmological observation of a series of cases and review of the literature. *Br J Ophthalmol.*, 2011, Jan, 95(1), 11-6.

[43] Fraitag, S; Rimella, A; de Prost, Y; Brousse, N; Hadj-Rabia, S; Bodemer, C. Skin biopsy is helpful for the diagnosis of incontinentia pigmenti at late stage (IV), a series of 26 cutaneous biopsies. *J Cutan Pathol.*, 2009, Sep, 36(9), 966-71.
[44] Charles, CR; Johnson, BL; Robinson, TA. Lichen striatus: a clinical, histologic and electron microscopic study of an unusual case. *J Cutan Pathol.*, 1974, 1(6), 265-74.
[45] Hauber, K; Rose, C; Brocker, EB; Hamm, H. Lichen striatus: clinical features and follow-up in 12 patients. *Eur J Dermatol.*, 2000, Oct-Nov, 10(7), 536-9.
[46] Hofer, T. Lichen striatus in adults or 'adult blaschkitis'?. There is no need for a new naming. *Dermatology.*, 2003, 207(1), 89-92.
[47] Patrizi, A; Neri, I; Fiorentini, C; Bonci, A; Ricci, G. Lichen striatus: clinical and laboratory features of 115 children. *Pediatr Dermatol.*, 2004, May-Jun, 21(3), 197-204.
[48] Taieb, A; el Youbi, A; Grosshans, E; Maleville, J. Lichen striatus: a Blaschko linear acquired inflammatory skin eruption. *J Am Acad Dermatol.*, 1991, Oct, 25(4), 637-42.
[49] Zhang, Y; McNutt, NS. Lichen striatus. Histological, immunohistochemical, and ultrastructural study of 37 cases. *J Cutan Pathol.*, 2001, Feb, 28(2), 65-71.
[50] Denk, K; Flux, K. Blaschkitis in children - a new entity? *J Dtsch Dermatol Ges.*, 2011, Jan, 9(1), 48-9.
[51] Keegan, BR; Kamino, H; Fangman, W; Shin, HT; Orlow, SJ; Schaffer, JV. "Pediatric blaschkitis": expanding the spectrum of childhood acquired Blaschko-linear dermatoses. *Pediatr Dermatol.*, 2007, Nov-Dec, 24(6), 621-7.
[52] Grosshans, E; Marot, L. [Blaschkitis in adults]. *Ann Dermatol Venereol.*, 1990, 117(1), 9-15.
[53] Muller, CS; Schmaltz, R; Vogt, T; Pfohler, C. Lichen striatus and blaschkitis: reappraisal of the concept of blaschkolinear dermatoses. *Br J Dermatol.*, 2011, Feb, 164(2), 257-62.
[54] Lee, SH; Rogers, M. Inflammatory linear verrucous epidermal naevi: a review of 23 cases. *Australas J Dermatol.*, 2001, Nov, 42(4), 252-6.
[55] Adrian, RM; Baden, HP. Analysis of epidermal fibrous proteins in inflammatory linear verrucous epidermal nevus. *Arch Dermatol.*, 1980, Oct, 116(10), 1179-80.
[56] Bernhard, JD; Owen, WR; Steinman, HK; Kaplan, LA; Menkes, AB; Baden, HP. Inflammatory linear verrucous epidermal nevus. Epidermal

protein analysis in four patients. *Arch Dermatol.*, 1984, Feb, 120(2), 214-5.

[57] de Jong, E; Rulo, HF; van de Kerkhof PC. Inflammatory linear verrucous epidermal naevus (ILVEN) versus linear psoriasis. A clinical, histological and immunohistochemical study. *Acta Derm Venereol.*, 1991, 71(4), 343-6.

[58] Hofer, T. Does inflammatory linear verrucous epidermal nevus represent a segmental type 1/type 2 mosaic of psoriasis? *Dermatology.*, 2006, 212(2), 103-7.

[59] Ito, M; Shimizu, N; Fujiwara, H; Maruyama, T; Tezuka, M. Histopathogenesis of inflammatory linear verrucose epidermal naevus: histochemistry, immunohistochemistry and ultrastructure. *Arch Dermatol Res.*, 1991, 283(8), 491-9.

[60] Oram, Y; Arisoy, AE; Hazneci, E; Gurer, I; Muezzinoglu, B; Arisoy, ES. Bilateral inflammatory linear verrucous epidermal nevus associated with psoriasis. *Cutis.*, 1996, Apr, 57(4), 275-8.

[61] Vissers, WH; Muys, L; Erp, PE; de Jong, EM; van de Kerkhof, PC. Immunohistochemical differentiation between inflammatory linear verrucous epidermal nevus (ILVEN) and psoriasis. *Eur J Dermatol.*, 2004, Jul-Aug, 14(4), 216-20.

[62] Patsatsi, A; Böer, A. Linear dermatoses—Part 2: Linear psoriasis, nevoid psoriasis, or inflammatory linear verrucous epidermal nevus (ILVEN)? *Dermatopathol Pract Conc*, 2010, 16(1), 4, 2010, 16(1)(4).

[63] Scott, LA; Stone, MS. Viral exanthems. *Dermatol Online J.*, 2003, Aug, 9(3), 4.

[64] Bohr-Nischal, U; Khopkar, U; Kharkar, V; Böer-Auer, A. New Insights: Lichen planus in children and adults. *Dermatopathol Prac Conc.*, 2010, 16(2)(3).

[65] Brockow, K; Abeck, D; Haupt, G; Ring, J. Exanthematous lichen planus in a child--response to acitretin. *Br J Dermatol.*, 1997, Feb, 136(2), 287-9.

[66] Handa, S; Sahoo, B. Childhood lichen planus: a study of 87 cases. *Int J Dermatol.*, 2002, Jul, 41(7), 423-7.

[67] Kanwar, AJ; De, D. Lichen planus in childhood: report of 100 cases. *Clin Exp Dermatol.*, 2010, Apr, 35(3), 257-62.

[68] Kumar, B; Kaur, I; Bhattacharya, M. Dapsone in lichen planus. *Acta Derm Venereol.*, 1994, Jul, 74(4), 334.

[69] Limas, C; Limas, CJ. Lichen planus in children: a possible complication of hepatitis B vaccines. *Pediatr Dermatol.*, 2002, May-Jun, 19(3), 204-9.

[70] Merigou, D; Leaute-Labreze, C; Louvet, S; Bioulac-Sage, P; Taieb, A. [Lichen planus in children: role of the campaign for hepatitis B vaccination]. *Ann Dermatol Venereol.*, 1998, Jul, 125(6-7), 399-403.

[71] Milligan, A; Graham-Brown, RA. Lichen planus in children--a review of six cases. *Clin Exp Dermatol.*, 1990, Sep, 15(5), 340-2.

[72] Nanda, A; Al-Ajmi, HS; Al-Sabah, H; Al-Hasawi, F; Alsaleh, QA. Childhood lichen planus: a report of 23 cases. *Pediatr Dermatol.*, 2001, Jan-Feb, 18(1), 1-4.

[73] Oono, T; Arata, J. Childhood lichen planus in a patient receiving growth hormone for dwarfism. *Dermatology.*, 1996, 192(1), 87-8.

[74] Rybojad, M; Moraillon, I; Laglenne, S; Vignon-Pennamen, MD; Bonvalet, D; Prigent, F; et al. [Lichen planus in children: 12 cases]. *Ann Dermatol Venereol.*, 1998, Oct, 125(10), 679-81.

[75] Sharma, R; Maheshwari, V. Childhood lichen planus: a report of fifty cases. *Pediatr Dermatol.*, 1999, Sep-Oct, 16(5), 345-8.

[76] Tasanen, K; Renko, M; Kandelberg, P; Herva, R; Oikarinen, A. Childhood lichen planus after simultaneous measles-mumps-rubella and diphtheria-tetanus-pertussis-polio vaccinations. *Br J Dermatol.*, 2008, Mar, 158(3), 646-8.

[77] Clayton, TH; Wilkinson, SM; Rawcliffe, C; Pollock, B; Clark, SM. Allergic contact dermatitis in children: should pattern of dermatitis determine referral? A retrospective study of 500 children tested between 1995 and 2004 in one U.K. centre. *Br J Dermatol.*, 2006, Jan, 154(1), 114-7.

[78] Czarnobilska, E; Obtulowicz, K; Dyga, W; Spiewak, R. A half of schoolchildren with 'ISAAC eczema' are ill with allergic contact dermatitis. *J Eur Acad Dermatol Venereol.*, 2011 Sep, 25(9), 1104-7.

[79] Milingou, M; Tagka, A; Armenaka, M; Kimpouri, K; Kouimintzis, D; Katsarou, A. Patch tests in children: a review of 13 years of experience in comparison with previous data. *Pediatr Dermatol.*, 2010, May-Jun, 27(3), 255-9.

[80] Shah, M; Lewis, FM; Gawkrodger, DJ. Patch testing in children and adolescents: five years' experience and follow-up. *J Am Acad Dermatol.*, 1997, Dec, 37(6), 964-8.

[81] Rajagopalan, R; Anderson, RT; Sarma, S; Kallal, J; Retchin, C; Jones, J; et al. An economic evaluation of patch testing in the diagnosis and management of allergic contact dermatitis. *Am J Contact Dermat.*, 1998, Sep, 9(3), 149-54.

[82] Hsu, JW; Matiz, C; Jacob, SE. Nickel allergy: localized, id, and systemic manifestations in children. *Pediatr Dermatol.*, 2011, May-Jun, 28(3), 276-80.
[83] McLean, L; Yewchuk, L; Israel, DM; Prendiville, JS. Acute onset of generalized pruritic rash in a toddler. Diagnosis: systemic allergic (contact) dermatitis to nickel from ingestion of metal coins. *Pediatr Dermatol.*, 2011, Jan-Feb, 28(1), 53-4.
[84] Garcia, E; Halpert, E; Rodriguez, A; Andrade, R; Fiorentino, S; Garcia, C. Immune and histopathologic examination of flea bite-induced papular urticaria. *Ann Allergy Asthma Immunol.*, 2004, Apr, 92(4), 446-52.
[85] Jordaan, HF; Schneider, JW. Papular urticaria: a histopathologic study of 30 patients. *Am J Dermatopathol.*, 1997, Apr, 19(2), 119-26.
[86] Raza, N; Lodhi, MS; Ahmed, S; Dar, NR; Ali, L. Clinical study of papular urticaria. *J Coll Physicians Surg Pak.*, 2008, Mar, 18(3), 147-50.
[87] Ben-Amitai, D; Hodak, E; Landau, M; Metzker, A; Feinmesser, M; David, M. Idiopathic palmoplantar eccrine hidradenitis in children. *Eur J Pediatr.*, 2001, Mar, 160(3), 189-91.
[88] Kluger, N; Moguelet, P; Khosrotehrani, K; Aractingi, S. Idiopathic recurrent palmoplantar hidradenitis: a case with late onset and long-lasting course. *Clin Exp Dermatol.*, 2007, Mar, 32(2), 217-8.
[89] Landau, M; Metzker, A; Gat, A; Ben-Amitai, D; Brenner, S. Palmoplantar eccrine hidradenitis: three new cases and review. *Pediatr Dermatol.*, 1998, Mar-Apr, 15(2), 97-102.
[90] Simon, M; Jr., Cremer, H; von den Driesch, P. Idiopathic recurrent palmoplantar hidradenitis in children. Report of 22 cases. *Arch Dermatol.*, 1998, Jan, 134(1), 76-9.
[91] Akcay, A; Akar, M; Oncel, MY; Kizilelma, A; Erdeve, O; Oguz, SS; et al. Hypercalcemia Due to Subcutaneous Fat Necrosis in a Newborn After Total Body Cooling. *Pediatr Dermatol.*, 2012, Feb 22.
[92] Akin, MA; Akin, L; Sarici, D; Yilmaz, I; Balkanli, S; Kurtoglu, S. Follow-up during early infancy of newborns diagnosed with subcutaneous fat necrosis. *J Clin Res Pediatr Endocrinol.*, 2011, 3(4), 216-8.
[93] Hogeling, M; Meddles, K; Berk, DR; Bruckner, AL; Shimotake, TK; Cohen, RS; et al. Extensive subcutaneous fat necrosis of the newborn associated with therapeutic hypothermia. *Pediatr Dermatol.*, 2012, Jan-Feb, 29(1), 59-63.
[94] Schubert, PT; Razack, R; Vermaak, A; Jordaan, HF. Fine-needle aspiration cytology of subcutaneous fat necrosis of the newborn: the

cytology spectrum with review of the literature. *Diagn Cytopathol.*, 2012, Mar, 40(3), 245-7.

[95] Grogg, KL; Nascimento, AG. Subcutaneous granuloma annulare in childhood: clinicopathologic features in 34 cases. *Pediatrics.*, 2001, Mar, 107(3), E42.

[96] Neto Pimentel, DR; Michalany, N; De Abreu, MA; Alchorne, M. Multiple deep granuloma annulare limited to the cephalic segment in childhood. *Pediatr Dermatol.*, 2008, May-Jun, 25(3), 407-8.

[97] Requena, L; Fernandez-Figueras, MT. Subcutaneous granuloma annulare. *Semin Cutan Med Surg.*, 2007, Jun, 26(2), 96-9.

[98] Stefanaki, K; Tsivitanidou-Kakourou, T; Stefanaki, C; Valari, M; Argyrakos, T; Konstantinidou, CV; et al. Histological and immuno-histochemical study of granuloma annulare and subcutaneous granuloma annulare in children. *J Cutan Pathol.*, 2007, May, 34(5), 392-6.

[99] Boer, A; Blodorn-Schlicht, N; Wiebels, D; Steinkraus, V; Falk, TM. Unusual histopathological features of cutaneous leishmaniasis identified by polymerase chain reaction specific for Leishmania on paraffin-embedded skin biopsies. *Br J Dermatol.*, 2006, Oct, 155(4), 815-9.

[100] Grech, V; Mizzi, J; Mangion, M; Vella, C. Visceral leishmaniasis in Malta--an 18 year paediatric, population based study. *Arch Dis Child.*, 2000, May, 82(5), 381-5.

[101] Pace, D; Williams, TN; Grochowska, A; Betts, A; Attard-Montalto, S; Boffa, MJ; et al. Manifestations of paediatric Leishmania infantum infections in Malta. *Travel Med Infect Dis.*, 2011, Jan, 9(1), 37-46.

[102] Martin-Ezquerra, G; Fisa, R; Riera, C; Rocamora, V; Fernandez-Casado, A; Barranco, C; et al. Role of Leishmania spp. infestation in nondiagnostic cutaneous granulomatous lesions: report of a series of patients from a Western Mediterranean area. *Br J Dermatol.*, 2009, Aug, 161(2), 320-5.

[103] Fraga, J; Veland, N; Montalvo, AM; Praet, N; Boggild, AK; Valencia, BM; et al. Accurate and rapid species typing from cutaneous and mucocutaneous leishmaniasis lesions of the New World. *Diagn Microbiol Infect Dis.*, 2012, Oct, 74(2), 142-50.

In: Dermatitis
Editor: Cornelia Sigrid Lissi Müller
ISBN: 978-1-62618-997-3

Chapter II

Dermatitis in Childhood – Causes and Treatment Options

Claudia Schiekofer *

The Saarland University Hospital, Department of Dermatology, Homburg/Saar, Germany

Abstract

Atopic dermatitis is the best-known type of dermatitis in infancy and childhood [1]; however, there are a number of other forms of dermatitis which appear during this period of life. For pediatric patients, these diseases cause physical symptoms, such as itching, pain, or burning of the skin. Even the development of children can be disturbed by dermatitis (e.g., insomnia resulting from pruritus) [2]. There can also be psychological problems associated with dermatitis (reaction of the environment and embarrassment). Children can be unkind to each other, especially based on differences in appearance!

This chapter specifically concentrates on the following most common types of dermatitis in infancy and childhood, as follows: atopic; seborrhoic; perioral; nummular; and contact (in particular, diaper dermatitis).

Also the chapter explains the causes and different treatment options for dermatitis. Each type of dermatitis has a typical time in life during

* Corresponding author: Phone: 0049-6841-16 23793, Fax: 0049-6841-16 23845, Email: claudia.schiekofer@uks.eu.

which it occurs. For example, it is unusual that a child < 5 years of age has nummular dermatitis [1]; however, atopic dermatitis can develop in early infancy. There is a great diversity in the management of the different forms of dermatitis. The use of steroids or antibiotics is not always preferred. There are relatively new products, such as tacrolimus (Protopic®) or pimecrolimus (Elidel®), which represent good alternatives to steroids for the treatment of dermatitis. Systemic therapy (e.g., antibiotics) in addition to external therapy is sometimes necessary.

Introduction

The best-known type of dermatitis in infancy and childhood is atopic dermatitis [1]; however, there are other forms of dermatitis which appear during this period of life. It is noteworthy that each type of dermatitis has its typical time in life during which it occurs [1].

This chapter aims to provide an overview of the most common types of dermatitis in childhood, the causes, and a selection of treatment options.

Atopic Dermatitis

Atopic dermatitis is the most well-known representative of dermatitis in infancy and childhood. Typically for atopic dermatitis are inflammatory lesions which are chronic or chronically recurring, and appear in different areas depending on patient age. In infancy there are preferred localizations to the face and extensors of the lower legs, while in childhood the flexures are typically affected [1]. Atopic dermatitis is also characterized by severe itching. In fact, itching is often the worst symptom for pediatric patients and their families.

The most common age of onset for atopic dermatitis is during the preschool years [2]. This period of life is characterized by important developments in psychosocial and physical behaviour, such as sleep patterns [3]. Children with atopic dermatitis often have reduced sleep efficiency caused by frequent awakenings, and daytime tiredness; thus, normal development and even normal family life can be disturbed. Children with atopic dermatitis are often described by their parents as being clingy, fearful, frustrated, and hyperactive [4]. Some parents of children with atopic dermatitis feel guilty, especially if they also have atopic dermatitis, and think that this is the reason that their child has the same disease. As a result, parents often change their lifestyle, such as a change in the home environment and planning other vacations and activities [4]. Often these changes create a financial burden [4], which in turn complicates the situation.

Epidemiology/Pathogenesis

Of the children living in northern Europe, 10%-20% are affected by atopic dermatitis [5].

The pathogenesis underlying atopic dermatitis is complex. There are interactions between the immune system, genetic, metabolic, infectious, and neuroendocrine factors, as well as the influence of the environment [6].

Clinical/Symptoms

There are some criteria that must be followed to diagnose atopic dermatitis (pruritus and eczema [acute, sub acute, or chronic]) (see Figure 1 and 2) [6]. The vast majority of patients or their families have an atopic background and xerosis cutis [6]. Furthermore, there are non-specific clinical associations to help diagnose atopic dermatitis, Such as white dermographism, facial pallor, or keratosis pilaris [6].

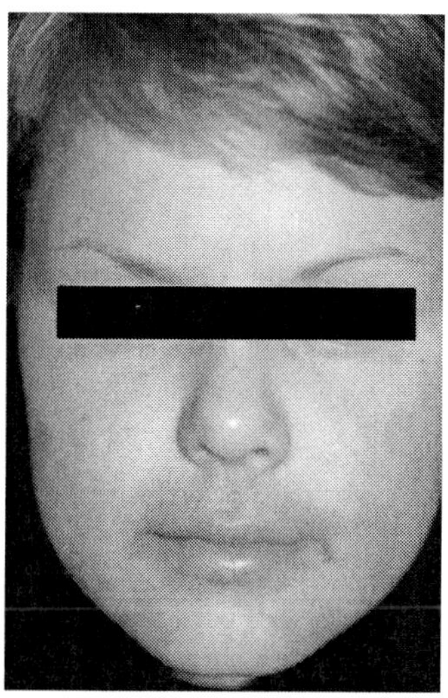

Figure 1. Atopic dermatitis revealing atopic stigmata.

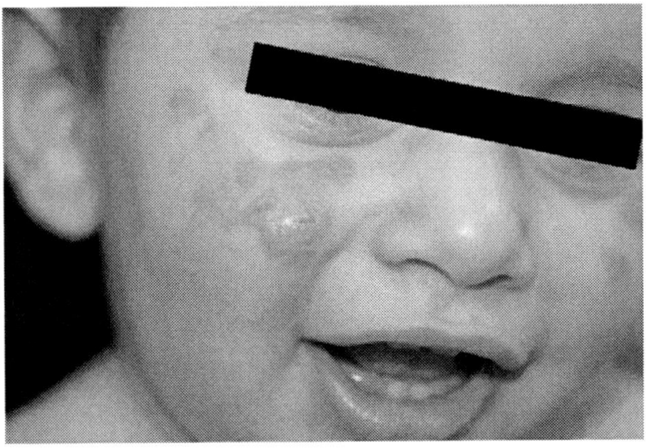

Figure 2. Atopic dermatitis in a baby.

Therapy

The treatment of atopic dermatitis is challenging because of number of local and systemic therapies are not allowed for children. There is no possibility to cure atopic dermatitis; only the symptoms can be treated or controlled [6].

There are general rules for behaviour amongst children with atopic dermatitis.

The parents should avoid clothes made from wool because of the irritant potential. Cotton clothes are preferred [5]. Also, other irritants, such as overheating or external irritants, are forbidden [6]. Emollients should be used for cleaning. The most commonly used local therapy substances for atopic dermatitis are corticosteroids [7]. Since the early 1950s, topical corticosteroids have been used with great success [8]. With respect to therapy of children, it is noteworthy that the risk of systemic absorption of topically applied corticosteroids relative to weight is increased [8]. Furthermore, one must consider the side effects of topical corticosteroids. There are only a few clinical studies available on the efficacy and safety of topical corticosteroids in young children with atopic dermatitis [9].

Other treatment options for atopic dermatitis include photo chemotherapy or systemic treatments, such as corticosteroids, cyclosporine, or azathioprine, all of which have relative contraindications in the therapy of children [10] and are often not thoroughly tested for this age group. In mild cases of atopic dermatitis, local treatment and adherence to general rules of behavior is often sufficient. If not enough sufficient, there is the possibility to use a local corticosteroid of low potential for as short a period as possible. Cortisone-free therapy is desired. One possibility to reduce the use of corticosteroids is the use of calcineurin inhibitors, such as pimecrolimus and tacrolimus. To treat children < 2 years of age with these substances is off-label use [6]. Because it is necessary to have a signed consent from parents, tacrolimus and pimecrolimus should be used as second-line therapy for moderate or severe atopic dermatitis [6].

Sometimes local therapy for atopic dermatitis in childhood is not adequate. There are different possibilities of systemic treatment for severe atopic dermatitis. One can give systemic corticosteroids, but there are known side such as suppression of the hypothalamic-pituitary-adrenal axis or growth [6]. A risk-benefit analysis should be performed before starting such therapy.

Because of the pruritus, one can administer anti-histamines, but to avoid daytime tiredness, anti-histamines should be given at bedtime [6].

In some cases there is also a secondary bacterial infection, often with *Staphylococcus aureus*. The treatment for secondary bacterial infections is typically antibiotics (local and systemic) [6].

Systemic immunomodulators, such as azathioprine, cyclosporine, and mycophenolate, are only used for severe forms of atopic dermatitis [6]. Thus far the availability of data has been poor with respect to the utility and safety of systemic immunomodulators in pediatrics [6].

Cyclosporine acts directly with an inhibitory effect on T cells [11]; however, adverse effects can appear during therapy with cyclosporine. The most frequent are adverse effects are hypertension and renal dysfunction, both of which are usually reversible after drug discontinuation [11]. Normally this kind of treatment is well-tolerated in children [11], but adequate studies are lacking [11]. If cyclosporine cannot be administered or there is an inadequate effect, other drugs should be tried, such as azathioprine [11]. There are case reports about the safety of azathioprine therapy in the treatment of infantile atopic dermatitis. Before starting therapy with azathioprine, the thiopurine methyltransferase activity should be checked [12].

Seborrhoic Dermatitis

Seborrhoic dermatitis of childhood is probably unrelated to the adult variant [1]. This form of dermatitis is frequently confused with atopic dermatitis, but there are notable differences in the clinical symptoms.

Epidemiology/Pathogenesis

It has been suggested that the childhood variant of seborrhoic dermatitis is caused by an overgrowth of *Pityrosporon ovale,* which is a yeast-like organism [13].

Clinical/Symptoms

Areas most affected in patients with seborrhoic dermatitis are the scalp, face, and flexures (see Figure 3) [1]. The eyebrows and nasolabial folds are often involved. Seborrhoic dermatitis usually begins soon after birth during the first 8 weeks of life [1].

Typically, oily and shiny scales, sometimes with an erythematous base, are observed [1]. These lesions on the head are sometimes referred to as "cradle cap" [1].

In contrast to atopic dermatitis, the scale is less dry, adherent, and rarely crusted; there is also less pruritus and rare hair loss [1]. "Infants with seborrhoic dermatitis may have extensive lesions, but are happy babies, while infants with atopic dermatitis are irritable and itchy" [1].

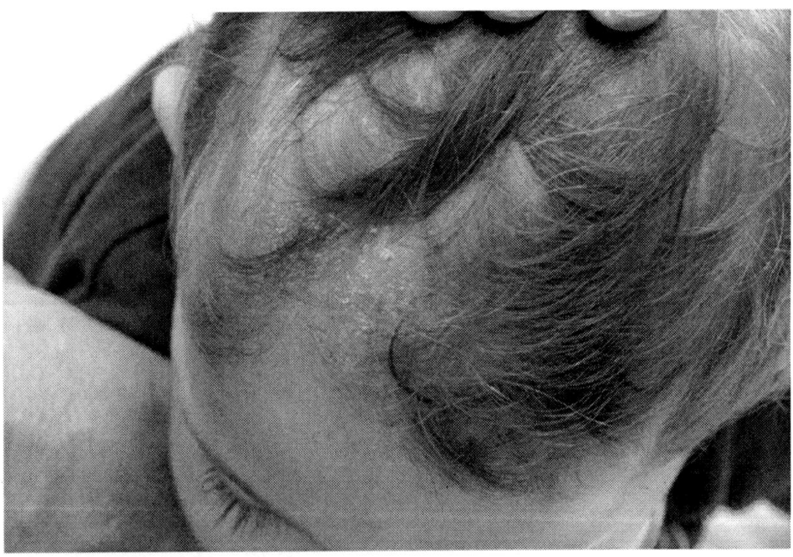

Figure 3. Seborrhoic scalp eczema.

Therapy

For infants with seborrhoic dermatitis, it is necessary to launder and change the diapers frequently. Occlusive clothing should be avoided. The scales can be peeled off with olive oil, when indicated, in combination with salicylic acid. If there are additional bacterial super infections the application of antibacterial substances is recommended. When the scales are peeled off, steroid-containing products can be used, but only for a short time. If there is a confirmed fungal infection of the skin, application of amphotericin B, nystatin, or imidazole should be considered. In most cases, systemic therapy is not necessary. Systemic steroids or antibiotics are reserved for severe cases.

Perioral Dermatitis

Perioral dermatitis starts later in life than atopic dermatitis [1]. In contrast to atopic dermatitis, perioral dermatitis is usually confined to the face [1].

Epidemiology/Pathogenesis

The epidemiology and pathogenesis underlying perioral dermatitis are not known; however, there appears to be a link between the appearance of perioral dermatitis and the use of topical corticosteroids, ointments, or creams [14]. Perioral dermatitis in children is also known as Gianotti-type perioral dermatitis, granulomatous perioral dermatitis of childhood, or rosacea-like eruption of children [14]. The adult form of perioral dermatitis and the childhood variant have many clinical symptoms in common [15].

Clinical/Symptoms

There are papular and acneiform lesions around the mouth that spares the vermillion border (Figure 4) [1, 14]. There are also vesicles or pustules [15]. The perinasal or periorbital area can be affected [14]. Typically, children otherwise have no remarkable systemic symptoms; even the pruritus is highly variable [14].

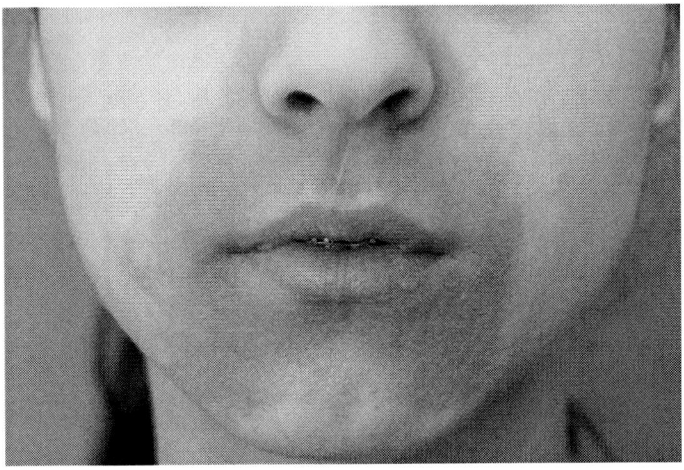

Figure 4. Classical appearance of perioral dermatitis.

Therapy

During treatment of perioral dermatitis, the use of topical corticosteroid-containing agents should be stopped [14]. In some cases, the application of 0.75% metronidazole cream induces healing [14]. The treatment can be affected alone or in combination with alternative agents, such as erythromycin [14]. Why there is an effect of metronidazole on perioral dermatitis in childhood is unclear [14]. Perhaps the effect is based on the anti-inflammatory, immunosuppressive, or antimicrobial actions [14].

In severe cases of perioral dermatitis, if local therapy is not adequate, the treatment can be complemented with a systemic antibiotic. For children > 9 years of age, tetracycline (250 mg twice a day) is described as effective. There is a contraindication to the use of tetracyclines in children < 8 years of age because of the discoloration effect on teeth [15]. For children < 9 years of age, erythromycin can be used at a dose of 30-40 mg/kg/day in two divided doses [14].

Nummular Dermatitis

Nummular dermatitis is one of the most common misdiagnosed atopic dermatitis [1]. This disease is unusual in children < 5 years of age [1].

Epidemiology/Pathogenesis

The epidemiology and pathogenesis underlying nummular dermatitis is unknown.

Clinical/Symptoms

There is no preferred location for nummular dermatitis on the body. In contrast to atopic dermatitis, the patient has no history of xerosis of the skin (Figure 5) [1]. The lesions are typically small, pruritic, follicular papules which can confluence in large plaques [1]. There is often exudation and crustification [1].

Therapy

This variant of dermatitis often demands the application of topical steroids and systemic antibiotics [1]. In some cases, an antibiogram should be performed before starting with systemic antibiotics. The use of antiseptic agents can support local therapy.

Contact Dermatitis

The appearance of contact dermatitis in childhood is unusual, but possible [1]. The most important reasons why children have less contact dermatitis than the adult population are the lack of exposure to potential allergens and an immature immune system [17]. The most frequent cause of contact dermatitis is licking the lips [1]. This phenomenon appears often in the winter months [1] because of dryer lips this time of year.

Epidemiology/Pathogenesis

The causes of contact dermatitis are irritants, such as saliva or other ingredients that are potentially allergenic [1]. It is worth mentioning nickel as the most common allergic reaction in infants [1].

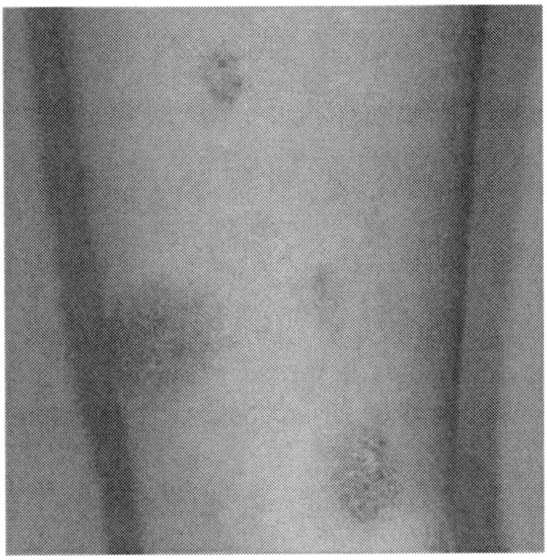

Figure 5. Nummular plaques at the extremities.

Clinical/Symptoms

The clinical symptoms of contact dermatitis are sometimes difficult to differentiate from the clinical symptoms of atopic dermatitis [1]. One of the leading symptoms in both diseases are severe pruritus [1]. To differentiate between atopic dermatitis and contact dermatitis it is often helpful to look after the affected areas (Figure 6). For example, if there is a contact reaction to nickel, areas in the midline of the chest are often involved because there are nickel snaps in undershirts [1]. Older children often have skin lesions, such as eczematous or lichenoid eruptions, just below the umbilicus because there are nickel snaps on the waistlines of jeans [1].

Also, to obtain a comprehensive medical history can help to differentiate between atopic dermatitis and contact dermatitis. The patients with contact dermatitis do not have xerosis under the skin like patients with atopic dermatitis [1].

Therapy

In treating contact dermatitis, it is important to removal all substances which can provoke the contact reaction [1]. The supporting use of topical steroids can be helpful, but it may take months for complete disappearance of the lesions [1].

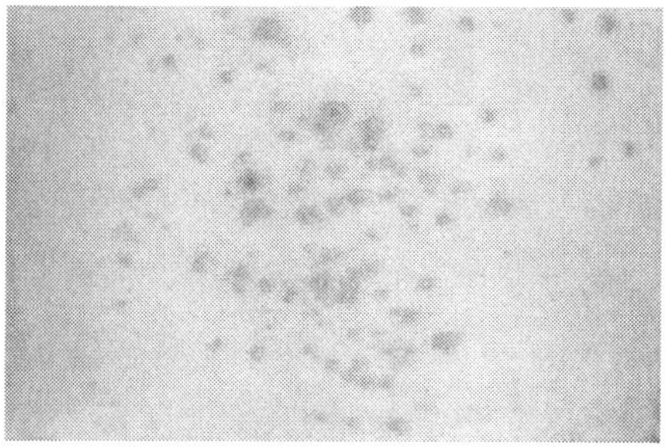

Figure 6. Typical primary efflorescence of acute contact dermatitis.

Conclusion

There are many different variants of dermatitis in childhood and infancy. There are many aspects to observe to establish the right diagnosis, as follows: the age of the patient when the first symptoms appear; the areas which are affected; the medical history of the child and the family; and any other systemic symptoms.

Therapy of all forms of dermatitis in childhood is a real challenge for every physician. In the literature there are only few studies which have investigated the treatment of dermatitis in childhood. Many therapies are contraindicated in children, such as systemic tetracyclines for children < 8 years of age [15]. Often the physician must analyze the risks and benefits of therapy, such as the use of corticosteroids.

References

[1] Krol, A; Krafchik, B. The differential diagnosis of atopic dermatitis in childhood. *Dermatol Ther*, 2006 Mar-Apr, 19(2), 73-82.

[2] Paller, AS; Chren, MM. Out of the skin of babes. Measuring the full impact of atopic dermatitis in infants and young children, *J Invest Dermatol*, 2012, 132, 2494–2496.

[3] Chamlin, SL; Chren, MM. Quality-of-life outcomes an measurement in childhood atopic dermatitis. *Immunol Allergy Clin North Am*, 30, 281-288.

[4] Chamlin, SL; Frieden, IJ; Williams, ML; et al. The effect of atopic dermatitis on young American children and their families. *Pediatrics.*, 2004, 114, 607-611.

[5] Schultz Larsen, F; Diepgen, T; Svensson, A. The occurrence of atopic dermtitis in North Europe: an international questionaire study. *J Am Acad Dermatol*, 1996, 34, 760-764.

[6] Eichenfield, LF; Hanifin, JM; Luer, TA; Stevens, SR; Pride, HB. Consensus conference on pediatric atopic dermatitis. *J Am Acad Dermatol*, 2003, 49, 1088-1095.

[7] Paller, AS; Nimmagadda, S; Schachner, L; Mallory, SB; Kahn, T; Willis, I; Eichenfield, F. Fluocinolone acetonide 0.01% in peanut oil: Therapy for childhood atopic dermatitis, even in patients who are peanut sensitve. *J AM Acad Dermatol*, 2003, 48, 569-577.

[8] Krafchik, BR. The use of topical steroids in children. *Semin Dermatol*, 1995, 14, 70-74.

[9] Wolkertorfer, A; Strobos, MA; Glazenburg, EJ; Mulder, PGH; Oranje, AP. Fluticasone proprionate 0.05% cream once daily versus clobetasone butyrate 0.05% cream twice daily in children with atopic dermatitis. *J AM Acad Dermatol*, 1998, 39, 226-231.

[10] Devillers, ACA; Oranje, AP. Wet-wrap treatment in children with atopic dermatitis: A practical guideline. *Pediatr Dermatol*, 2012, 29, 24-27.

[11] Ricci, G; Dondi, A; Patrizi, A; Masi, M. Systemic therapy of atopic dermatitis in children. *Drugs*, 2009, 69(3), 297-306.

[12] Martel, RM; Melwani, P; Islas, D; Penate, Y; Borrego, L. Safety of azathioprine therapy adjusted to thiopurine methyltransferase activity in the treatment of infantile atopic dermatitis. Report on 7 cases. *Actas Dermosifiliogr.*, 2012, 101 (5), 415-420.

[13] Zeharia, A; Mimouni, M; Fogel, D. Treatment with bifonazole shampoo for scalp seborrhoea in infants an young children. *Paediatr Dermatol*, 1996, 13, 151-153.

[14] Laude, TA; Salvemini, JN. Perioral dermatitis in children. *Semin Cutan Med Surg.*, 1999, (Sep), 18 (3), 206-209

[15] Manders, SM; Lucky, AW. Perioral dermatitis in childhood. *J AM Dermatol*, 1992, 27, 688-692

[16] Sharma, VK; Asati, DP. Pediatric contact dermatitis. *Indian J Dermatol Venerol Leprol*, 2010, 76, 514-520

In: Dermatitis
Editor: Cornelia Sigrid Lissi Müller
ISBN: 978-1-62618-997-3

Chapter III

Refutation of a Myth: Elastophagocytosis Is Not a Defining Criterion of Distinct Dermatoses

Cornelia S. L. Müller*

The Saarland University Hospital, Department of Dermatology, Homburg/ Saar, Germany

Abstract

Elastophagocytosis is used commonly to discriminate histologic findings for diverse dermatologic conditions, such as annular elastolytic giant cell granuloma or mid-dermal-elastolysis. This chapter was designed to identify the occurrence of elastophagocytosis in common granulomatous diseases to evaluate its impact. Three typical cases of mid dermal elastolysis with prominent elastophagocytosis and are shown and its relevancy is discussed. Additionally, the frequency of elastophagocytosis and fragmentation of elastic fibers in biopsies of granuloma annulare [GA] (n=11), cutaneous sarcoidal granulomatous inflammation [CSGI] (n=8), and lupoid rosacea [LR] (n=7), were retrospectively reviewed. Up to two-thirds of all cases of GA and CSGI

* Corresponding author: Phone: 0049-6841-16-23795, Fax: 0049-6841-16 13816, E-mail: cornelia.mueller@uks.eu.

investigated were characterized by elastophagocytosis. No dependence on chronic sun exposure was found. In summary, elastophagocytosis must be considered as a secondary cutaneous reaction pattern seen in any type of granulomatous inflammation and cannot be used as a defining criterion for histopathologic discrimination between distinct dermatologic entities.

Introduction

Elastophagocytosis (EP) is commonly defined as phagocytosis of distorted elastin by multinucleated giant cells. It is considered as a rather nonspecific finding in many different inflammatory diseases, and may also occur as a tumor-related phenomenon [1]. Conflicting data exist on the frequency of this phenomenon in various conditions. However, on the other hand, elastophagocytosis is seen as a defining criterion for specific diseases as annular elastolytic giant cell granuloma and mid dermal elastolysis. So particular, some granulomatous conditions exist, where elastophagocytosis is seen as a specific feature. Intriguingly, influence of chronic UV exposure, delayed-type hypersensitivity reaction, and secretion of diverse factors for activation and inactivation of macrophages and the release of proinflammatory cytokines have been implicated in the induction of elastophagocytosis [2-4]. However, the role of elastophagocytosis as a diagnostic criterion remains unclear. In this manuscript we do a dual approach pointing out the concept of elastophagocytosis by describing the clinical and histopathological features of three patients with the classical elastophagocytic dermatoses, mid-dermal elastolysis. In a second step we determine the frequency of elastophagocytosis and fragmentation of elastic fibers in biopsies of common granulomatous diseases such as granuloma annulare, cutaneous sarcoidal granulomatous inflammation, and lupoid rosacea, to verify its relevance for diagnosis as well as discuss its pathogenetic background.

Patients

The three patients presented were evaluated in our department between 2009 and 2011. Two of the three patients were male; the age of onset was between 5th and 6th decade. All patients displayed lesions in chronically sun-exposed areas and showed similar morphological findings of ringlike and annular macules associated with burning and itching sensations to a variable degree (Figure 1). Laboratory findings were inconclusive and light microscopy as well as cultures of the scales were negative for fungi in all three cases.

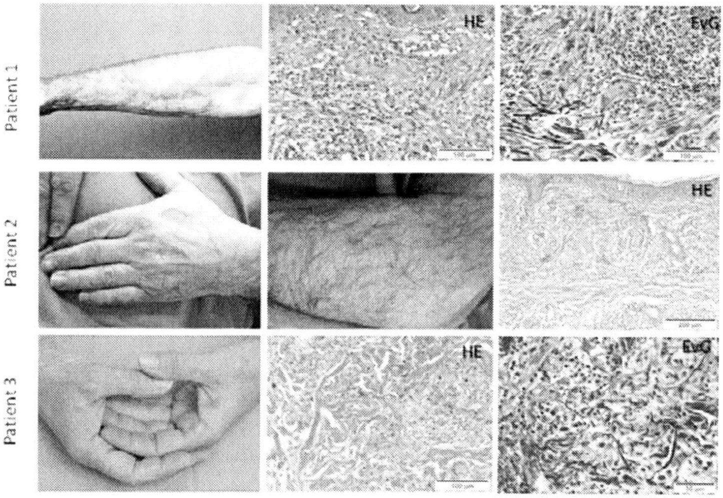

Figure 1. Distinct erythematous ring like macules on varying skin sites. Note, all areas are chronically sun damaged skin sites. Histomorphology on HE sections and elastophagocytosis in the presented cases.

Patient 1: A 57-year-old man presented with progressive erythematous-violaceous, sometimes ringlike somtimes reticulated macules associated with slight burning sensations, located symmetrically on forearms and back of the hands. Skin lesions started approximately two month before and had not been previously treated.

Patient 2: A 63-year-old male patient showed similar, on the back of the hands ringlike, on the forearms reticulated asymptomatic maculae with elevated papulous borders. Lesions first appeared three years before.

Patient 3: A 55-year-old female patient presented with erythematous annular papules on the skin between thumb and index finger, first appearing three months before on left hand, afterwards on right hand. Treatment with topical steroids had been performed and showed no evident benefit.

In all three cases, skin biopsies were taken from representative sites. We observed a normal epidermal band was seen with variable subepidermal inflammatory infiltrate. Strikingly, numerous of histiocytes, with one or more nuclei could be found in the mid dermis with a remarkable degree of elastophagocytosis and fragmentation and degeneration of elastic tissue. Surrounding tissue showed actinic damage (Figure 1).

Table 1a. Clinicopathologic data of patients with granuloma annulare

	clinical data			histopathological features (of elastic fibers)				
number	**age**	**gender**	**site**	**elastophagocytosis**	**deminishment**	**truncation**	**fragmentation**	**raveling**
1	39	m	lower right leg	positive	positive	positive	positive	not seen
2	50	m	back of the hand, right	positive	positive	positive	not seen	not seen
3	49	m	elbow right	positive	positive	positive	positive	not seen
4	75	f	left thigh	not seen	positive	positive	not seen	not seen
5	58	f	back of the hand, right	positive	positive	positive	positive	not seen
6	63	m	back of the hand, right	not seen	positive	positive	not seen	not seen
7	31	f	left groin	positive	not seen	not seen	positive	not seen
8	63	m	left knee	positive	positive	positive	positive	not seen
9	65	f	lower right leg	positive (esp. In active margins)	positive	positive	positive	not seen
10	55	f	not known	positive	not seen	not seen	not seen	not seen
11	69	f	left forearm	positive (esp. In active margins)	positive	not seen	not seen	not seen

Material and Methods

Histological Investigation

Tissue samples from 11 patients with granuloma annulare, 8 patients with cutaneous sarcoidal granulomatous inflammation, and seven patients with lupoid rosacea were analyzed retrospectively. All specimens were fixed in 4% neutral buffered formalin, processed routinely, and embedded in paraffin. For further investigations, sections were stained with Hematoxylin-eosin and an Elastica van Giesson's stain was performed.

The following histopathologic features were evaluated: presence of elastophagocytosis, diminishment, truncation, and fragmentation of elastic fibers.

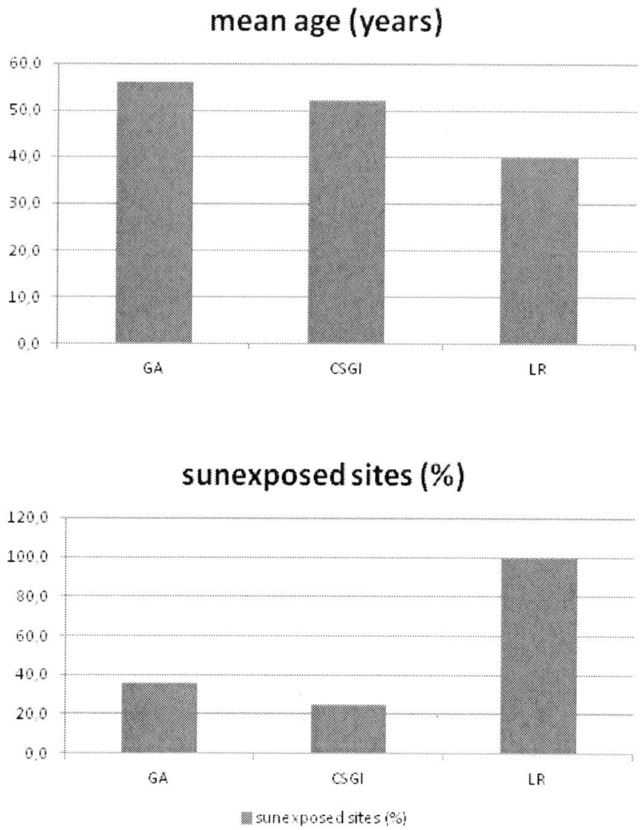

Figure 2a. Clinical data.

Study Population

Clinical data were obtained from patient charts and from referring physicians. Clinical data included age, sex, and site of disease. Data for individual patients enrolled in this study are shown in tables 1a-c. Twenty-six patients were included in this study (12 men and 14 women) with the following diagnoses: granuloma annulare (n=11); cutaneous sarcoidal granulomatous inflammation (n=8); and lupoid rosacea (n=7). Within the group of cutaneous sarcoidal granulomatous inflammation, sarcoidal reaction to implanted tattoo colors (n=3), scar sarcoidosis (n=1), granulomatous reaction to surgical suture material after tumor excision (n=2), and cutaneous lesions of systemical sarcoidosis (n=2) were included.

Results

Clinical features of the 26 patients (14 women and 12 men) are summarized in Table 1-c.

Granuloma Annulare

This group included six women (54.5%) and five men (45.4%), with a mean age of 56.1 years (range from 31 to 75 years). Four of the 11 patients displayed lesions in chronically sun-exposed skin (back of the hand and forearm). Elastophagocytosis and diminishment of elastic fibers were seen in 9 of the 11 (81.8%), truncation of elastic fibers was found in eight of the 11 (72.7%), and fragmentation in six of the 11 (54.5%) among all cases of granuloma annulare investigated (Table 1a, Figure 4a).

Cutaneous Sarcoidal Granulomatous Inflammation

Among the patients in this group, the mean age was 52.2 years (range from 30 to 77 years). Three patients experienced sarcoidal reaction to implanted tattoo colors, one patient had scar sarcoidosis, two patients experienced a granulomatous reaction to surgical suture material after tumor excision, and two patients had cutaneous lesions in the setting of systemic sarcoidosis. Five of the eight patients (62.5%) were men and three of the eight were women (37.5%). Only three out of the eight lesions (37.5%) were seen in chronically sun-damaged skin (forearm, forehead, and back of the hand). Elastophagocytosis was observed in six of eight cases (75%), diminishment of elastic fibers was seen in seven of eight (87.6%), truncation of elastic fibers was found in three of eight (37.5%), and fragmentation in one of eight (12.5%) cases (Table 1b).

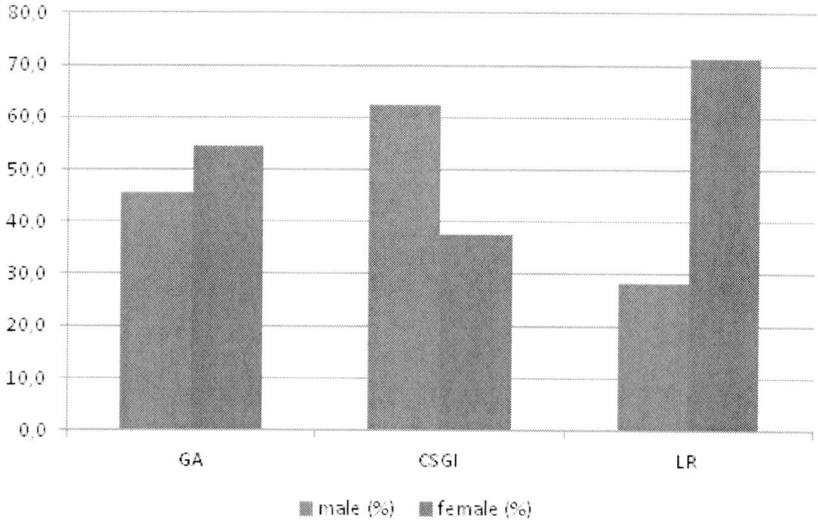

Figure 2b. Gender distribution (GA: granuloma annulare; CSGI: cutaneous sarcoidal granulomatous inflammation; LR: lupoid rosacea).

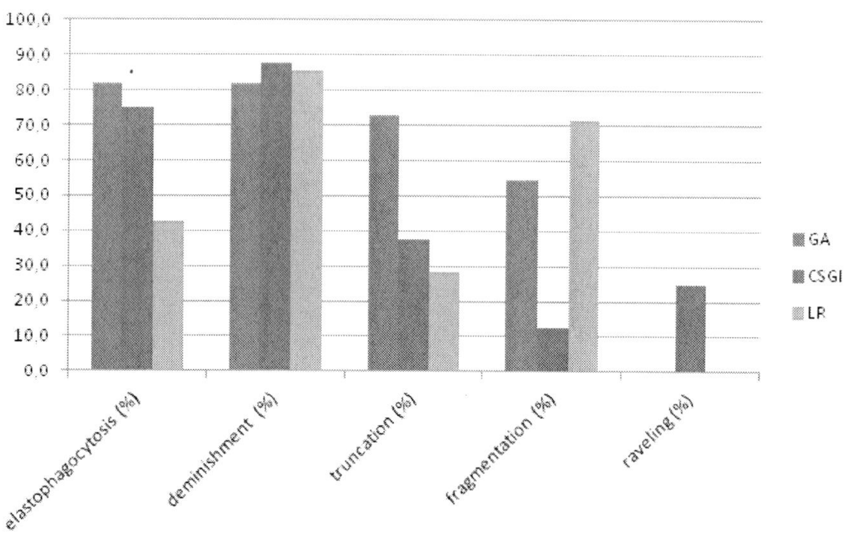

Figure 3. Histomorphological features of elastic fiber alteration.

Table 1b. Clinicopathologic data of patients with cutaneous sarcoidal granulomatous inflammation (CSGI)

	clinical data				histopathological features of (elastic fibers)				
No.	age	Gender	site	specials	Elastophagocytosis	Deminishment	Truncation	Fragmentation	Raveling
1	40	m	back		not seen	positive	not seen	not seen	not seen
2	34	f	left ankle	reaction to tattoo colour	positive	positive	not seen	not seen	not seen
3	30	f	left shoulder	reaction to tattoo colour	positive	positive	not seen	not seen	not seen
4	71	m	left forearm	scar sarcoidosis	positive	not seen	not seen	not seen	not seen
5	74	f	left shoulder	reaction to surgical suture material after excision of CTCL	positive	positive	positive	not seen	not seen
6	34	m	left knee	systemical sarcoidosis	not seen	positive	positive	not seen	not seen
7	77	m	facial, paranasal	reaction to surgucal suture material after excision of BCC	positive	positive	not seen	not seen	not seen
8	58	m	forehead	systemical sarcoidosis	positive	positive	positive	positive	Positive

Lupoid Rosacea

Mean age of patients with lupoid/ granulomatous rosacea was 40.1 years (range from 26 to 67 years). Five of the seven patients (71.4%) were women and two of the seven (28.5%) were men. Elastophagocytosis was observed in three of the seven cases (42,8%), diminishment of elastic fibers was seen in six of the seven (85,7%), truncation of elastic fibers was found in two of the seven (28.5%), and fragmentation in five of the seven (71.4%) (Table 1c). According to the definition of rosacea, all seven patients (100%) had lesions in chronically sun-damaged areas (face).

Discussion

The most important finding of this study is that the occurrence of elastophagocytosis is a frequent and fairly consistent finding in common granulomatous diseases and may therefore not be helpful to define the specific underlying setting.

Elastophagocytosis (EP) is commonly defined as phagocytosis of degenerated elastin by multinucleated giant cells [2, 5] (Figures 3, 4b). It is a non-specific finding in many different inflammatory diseases, but also is known as a tumor-related phenomenon [1, 6]. Dermatologic conditions exists in which elastophagocytosis is considered a defining feature. Actinic granuloma O`Brien [AG], annular elastolytic giant cell granuloma [AEGCG] and mid-dermal elastolysis (MDE) are the main conditions in this group [7]. Clinically, AG and AEGCG are similar and characteristically occur in both sun-damaged and sun-protected skin. But, the role of chronic UV exposure in the development of these diseases, especially in elastophagocytosis, is controversial [7-8], although these diseases mostly affect chronically sun damaged skin. Granuloma annulare is a common granulomatous disease characterized by a varying degree of palisaded granulomata and mucin deposition (Figure 4a). Intriguingly, UV light is not considered as a causal factor in pathogenesis of granuloma annulare. Disagreement exists about whether AG and AEGCG are subentities within the spectrum of GA, even though Limas argued for distinctive histomorphologic criteria that separate them from GA, such as the absence of connective tissue necrobiosis and changes in elastic tissue [7]. Hybrid lesions of AG and AEGCG have been described as the co-occurrence of two independent diseases as well as the manifestations of overlapping diseases [7-10].

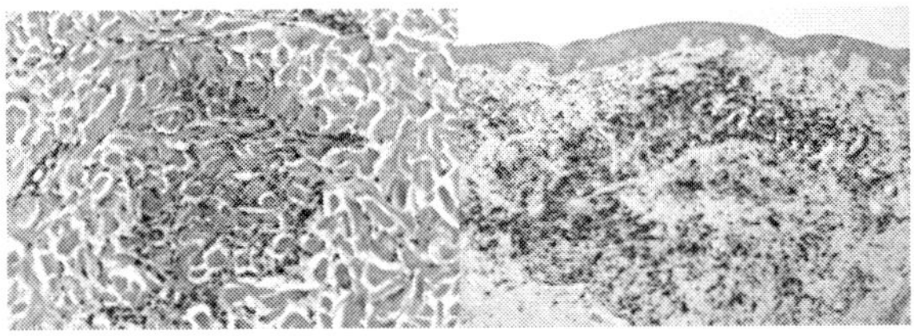

Figure 4a. Characteristic morphologic findings in fully developed granuloma annulare with palisaded granuloma and central necrobiosis. Left: HE stain, magnification 200x; right: CD68 stain displaying the granulomatous infiltrate forming palisaded granulomas, magnification 200x.

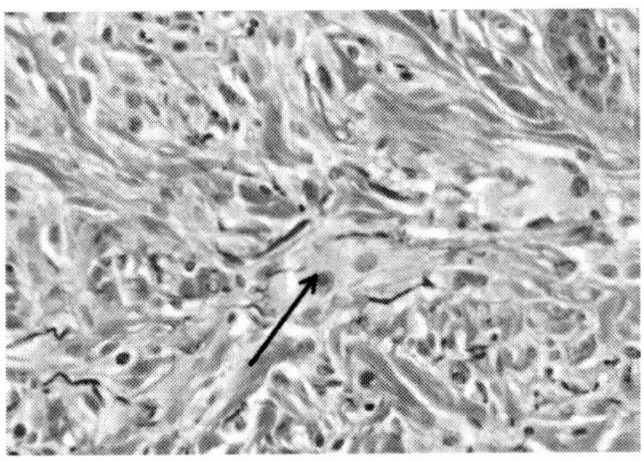

Figure 4b. Phagocytosis of altered elastic fibers by multinucleated giant cells, Elastica Van Giesson's stain, magnification 600x.

However, the diagnostic significance and frequency of elastophagocytosis have not been investigated on a larger scale. Furthermore, the nomenclature used to describe the quantitative morphologic or qualitative changes in elastic fiber composition and appearance related to elastophagocytosis is not consistent. Elastophagocytosis is consistently found – to varying degrees – in the cases of GA, LR, and CSGI investigated in this study. Within the CSGI group, distinct clinical findings were included, displaying all elastotic material within histiocytes. These results disagree with those of Al-Hoqail et al. who reported that no GA-biopsies displayed elastophagocytosis, and those of Günes et al. who reported elastophagocytosis in only 2 of 38 cases of GA [2, 11]. These differing results could be due to the lack of detection of elastophagocytosis, if diagnoses are made focusing on palisaded granulomas with mucin deposition in the upper dermis in conventional HE sections. Some other groups also found elastophagocytosis to varying degree in up to 100% of all cases investigated [12-15]. For that reason, Elastica van Giesson's stains are mandatory in this setting.

Table 1c. Clinicopathologic data of patients with lupoid/ granulomatous rosacea (LR)

	clinical data			histopathological features				
number	**age**	**gender**	**site**	**elastophagocytosis**	**deminishment**	**truncation**	**fragmentation**	**raveling**
1	55	f	facial	positive	positive	not seen	positive	not seen
2	26	f	facial	not seen	positive	positive	positive	not seen
3	67	f	facial	positive	positive	not seen	positive	not seen
4	29	m	facial	not seen	positive	not seen	not seen	not seen
5	39	f	facial	not seen	positive	positive	positive	not seen
6	46	m	facial	positive	positive	not seen	positive	not seen
7	19	f	facial	not seen	not seen	not seen	not seen	not seen

Elastophagocytosis appears in granulomatous inflammatory infiltrates as well as in non-granulomatous conditions, prompting discussion about whether it is an incidental finding of activated histiocytes [7]. Intriguingly, elastophagocytosis is observed in the surrounding of cutaneous neoplasms [1]. Sweeney and McDermott reported (1996) that elastophagocytosis was present in 77% of atypical fibroxanthomas investigated. However, only 6% of epithelial tumors exhibited elastophagocytosis [1]. They proposed that atypical fibroxanthoma influences surrounding cells and stroma to create an environment "responsible for modulating the non-specific inflammatory reaction, thereby inducing elastophagocytosis" [1]. Elastophagocytosis is found in chronic sun-exposed and in non-sun-exposed skin areas in younger as well as older persons. Ackerman (1979) reported that as a rule a granulomatous reaction is induced in sun-exposed skin, which leads to degeneration of elastic fibers with subsequent phagocytosis by histiocytic cell elements [9]. Our results support the findings of Günes et al. that elastophagocytosis is a common secondary event for local tissue clearance and occurs independently of gender or age [2]

Existing pathogenetic theories differ on what occurs first – elastic tissue damage with consecutive elastophagocytosis or the reverse. Mackiewicz et al. showed that macrophages are involved in clearance of massive local cell and tissue necrosis and form multinucleated giant cells with subsequent formation of granulomas in pulmonary, nasopharyngeal, and cutaneous tissue of Wegener's granulomatosis [16]. Necrotic or apoptotic tissues release a variety of signaling factors that recruit phagocytes to the region in the skin by acting as chemoattractants (17). In addition, several membrane-bound proteins expressed on the surface of apoptotic cells can distinguish them from vital cells [17]. In Wegener's disease, macrophages cannot eliminate all of the necrotic and apoptotic tissue and still contain undigested cells and tissue particles. Mackiewicz et al. proposed that this remaining tissue induces formation of giant cell granulomas and leads to active local antigen processing and presentation [16]. This may also be true for elastophagocytosis. Locally altered elastic fibers in diverse skin diseases may express "location" signals that attract phagocytes, induce formation of every type of granuloma (palisaded, foreign body, sarcoidal), and serve as persisting phagocytosis-inducing factors during inflammation.

Similarly, AEGCG and MDE are usually affecting chronically sun exposed areas, so – according to Ackerman - due to the degree of UV damage liberation of elastotic material is initiated causing prominent elastophagocytosis, that by the way characterizes these dermatologic conditions.

In turn, even if elastophagocytosis is thought to be not a specific morphologic sign, we have to admit, that distinct conditions exist, that are characterized by a high degree of elastophagocytosis, as in the presented cases of annular elastolytic giant cell granuloma. Thus, it seems to be more a question of quantity than quality, whether elastophagocytosis can be accepted as a defining morphologic feature.

Especially if chronically sun damaged skin is affected, a condition that leads to massive liberation of elastotic material consecutive prominent elastophagocytosis can serve as one characterizing feature.

In conclusion, elastophagocytosis is a striking cutaneous reaction pattern seen in all types of granulomatous inflammation and cannot be used alone to discriminate histopathologically among distinct dermatologic entities, but serves as a supporting feature in distinct settings associated with severe chronically sun damage.

References

[1] Sweeney, EC; McDermott, M. Tumour related cutaneous elastophagocytosis. *J Clin Pathol.*, 1996, Jan, 49(1), 81-3.

[2] Gunes, P; Goktay, F; Mansur, AT; Koker, F; Erfan, G. Collagen-elastic tissue changes and vascular involvement in granuloma annulare: a review of 35 cases. *J Cutan Pathol.*, 2009, Aug, 36(8), 838-44.

[3] Stefanaki, K; Tsivitanidou-Kakourou, T; Stefanaki, C; Valari, M; Argyrakos, T; Konstantinidou, CV; et al. Histological and immuno-histochemical study of granuloma annulare and subcutaneous granuloma annulare in children. *J Cutan Pathol.*, 2007, May, 34(5), 392-6.

[4] Vaalamo, M; Kariniemi, AL; Shapiro, SD; Saarialho-Kere, U. Enhanced expression of human metalloelastase (MMP-12) in cutaneous granulomas and macrophage migration. *J Invest Dermatol.*, 1999, Apr, 112(4), 499-505.

[5] Loo, WJ; Rytina, E; Banfield, C. Elastophagocytosis: a feature of resolving Sweet's syndrome. *J Eur Acad Dermatol Venereol.*, 2004, Jul, 18(4), 471-3.

[6] Wong, T; Swain, F; Calonge, E. Nicorandil-associated perianal ulceration with prominent elastophagocytosis and flexural ulceration. *Br J Dermatol.* 2005, Jun, 152(6), 1360-1.

[7] Limas, C. The spectrum of primary cutaneous elastolytic granulomas and their distinction from granuloma annulare: a clinicopathological analysis. *Histopathology*., 2004 Mar, 44(3), 277-82.

[8] Revenga, F; Rovira, I; Pimentel, J; Alejo, M. Annular elastolytic giant cell granuloma--actinic granuloma? *Clin Exp Dermatol*., 1996, Jan, 21(1), 51-3.

[9] Ragaz, A; Ackerman, AB. Is actinic granuloma a specific condition? *Am J Dermatopathol*., 1979, Spring, 1(1), 43-50.

[10] Steffen, C. Actinic granuloma (O'Brien). *J Cutan Pathol*., 1988 Apr, 15(2), 66-74.

[11] Al-Hoqail, IA; Al-Ghamdi, AM; Martinka, M; Crawford, RI. Actinic granuloma is a unique and distinct entity: a comparative study with granuloma annulare. *Am J Dermatopathol*., 2002, Jun, 24(3), 209-12.

[12] Burket, JM; Zelickson, AS. Intracellular elastin in generalized granuloma annulare. *J Am Acad Dermatol*., 1986, Jun, 14(6), 975-81.

[13] Friedman-Birnbaum, R; Weltfriend, S; Kerner, H; Lichtig, C. Elastic tissue changes in generalized granuloma annulare. *Am J Dermatopathol*., 1989, Oct, 11(5), 429-33.

[14] Hanna, WM; Moreno-Merlo, F; Andrighetti, L. Granuloma annulare: an elastic tissue disease? Case report and literature review. *Ultrastruct Pathol*., 1999, Jan-Feb, 23(1), 33-8.

[15] Wolff, HH; Maciejewski, W. The ultrastructure of granuloma annulare. *Arch Dermatol Res*., 1977, Sep 27, 259(3), 225-34.

[16] Mackiewicz, Z; Rimkevicius, A; Petersen, J; Andersen, CB; Dudek, E; Vytrasova, M; et al. Macrophages overloaded with tissue debris in Wegener's granulomatosis. *Ann Rheum Dis*., 2005, Aug, 64(8), 1229-32.

[17] Flannagan, RS; Jaumouille, V; Grinstein, S. The Cell Biology of Phagocytosis. *Annu Rev Pathol*., 2011, Jan 25.

In: Dermatitis
Editor: Cornelia Sigrid Lissi Müller
ISBN: 978-1-62618-997-3

Chapter IV

Dermatitis and Mosaicism: Current Aspects on Apparent Genetic Events

Rebecca Körner*

The Saarland University Hospital, Department of Dermatology, Homburg/ Saar, Germany

Abstract

A genetic mosaicism denotes the presentation of two or more populations of cells with different genotypes in one individual who developed from a single fertilized egg. Genetic and epigenetic mosaicisms can be distinguished; the latter are caused by inactivation of genes by retrotransposons or by inactivation of the X-chromosome (Lyon hypothesis).

In the skin, mosaicism usually follows one of six different patterns: the Blaschko-linear pattern with small or broad lines, checkerboard pattern, phylloid pattern, lateralization pattern, and patchy pattern without midline separation. Blaschko-linear patterns are the most common; they are derived from the growth pattern of embryonic cells caused by alteration between longitudinal and horizontal growth. Some dermatoses follow Blaschko linear patterns; for example, incontinentia pigmenti,

* Corresponding author: Phone: 0049-6841-16-23806, Fax: 0049-6841-16 23845, E-mail: rebecca.koerner@uks.eu.

hypomelanosis of Ito, and also lichen striatus, blaschkitis or the inflammatory linear verrucous epidermal nevus (ILVEN).

Furthermore, a variety of dermatoses that usually affect the whole skin also manifest in a segmental pattern; segmental type-I and type-II manifestation can be distinguished whereas the latter reflects a loss of heterozygosity.

For epidermal nevus syndromes, cutaneous mosaicisms may be the initial indication of a systemic disease, such as blaschko-linear nevus sebaceous in Schimmelpenning-Feuerstein-Mims-syndrome.

Introduction

A mosaic is comprised of differing components, such as differently colored stones. In genetics, the term mosaicism denotes the presentation of two or more populations of cells with different genotypes in one individual who has developed from a single fertilized egg. Because the skin can easily be seen, in contrast to other organs, the skin is in a unique position for the study of mosaicism.

Alfred Blaschko, in 1901, was the first to observe that some dermatoses follow certain cutaneous lines [1]. He described lines that formed a bizarre fountain-like pattern on the back, whorls on the abdomen, and linear stripes on the limbs.

Many nevoid and genetic skin diseases follow these lines [1]. He also observed that these lines were not related to the distribution of the nerves in the skin, and hypothesized an embryonic origin. However, it was not for another 75 years until Jackson in 1976 suggested a chromosomal mosaicism as the cause of the Blaschko lines [2].

However, he could not prove his hypothesis. In 1976, Rudolf Happle linked the lines of Blaschko to X-inactivation [3].

Development of Cutaneous Mosaicism

Two major subtypes of mosaicism can be distinguished: genomic and functional (epigenetic) mosaicism [4].

Genomic Mosaicism

Genomic mosaicism is caused by true mutations in which alterations in the DNA-sequence affect chromosomes and/or genes and a genetically heterogeneous organism develops.

Mutations may occur as:

A. Half-Chromatid Mutation in a Gamete

Deficient DNA replication in one single strand can cause mutation in a gamete. After fertilization, a chromosome with two different chromatids results due to semi-conservative replication. When the zygote divides in two, genetically different cells result. This can lead to an extensive mosaicism, such as, for example, systematized epidermal nevus.

B. Postzygotic Mutations

Postzygotic mutations are the simplest cause of a cutaneous mosaic. The earlier the mutation takes place in embryogenesis, the more skin will be affected.

C. Postzygotic Lethal Mutations

Some mutations are viable only as a mosaicism with a normal cell population. If the mutation is passed on to the zygote it will not survive. Some examples of lethal mutations are Schimmelpenning-Feuerstein-Mims syndrome or McCune-Albright syndrome.

D. Revertant Mosaicism (Back-Mutation)

Revertant mosaicism was first described in Lesch-Nyhan syndrome in 1988 [7]. It is a phenomenon that may occur in autosomal recessive skin diseases; postzygotic back-mutation areas of non affected skin can be observed in Epidermolysis bullosa or Ichthyosis variegata, for example.

E. Paradominant Inheritance

Paradominant inheritance is caused by loss of heterozygosity, a genetic mechanism in which a heterozygous somatic cell becomes either homozygous or hemizygous because the corresponding wild-type allele is lost [8]. This mechanism potentially explains the exceptional familial occurrence of nevi, such as in melanosis naeviformis. Heterozygote gene carriers are healthy and therefore the mutation is passed on from generation to generation. The disease manifests as a mosaicism only if loss of heterozygosity occurs during an early state of embryogenesis.

Epigenetic Mosaicism

Epigenetic mosaicism is a functional mosaic, which means that all cells have the same chromosomal set but may differ in their function. Changes in gene expression are passed on from one cell generation to the next but do not entail an alteration in the DNA-sequence [5]. The following changes are distinguishable:

A. X-Chromosomal Mosaicism

Lyonization, the random inactivation of one of the two x-chromosomes in each cell during early development (at approximately 1000-cell stage) of female embryos, is an important example of functional mosaicism [6]. Thus, all females are functionally mosaic. Incontinentia pigmenti, CHILD syndrome, and MIDAS syndrome are examples of dermatoses caused by x-chromosomal inactivation.

B. Autosomal Mosaicism

In autosomal mosaicism genes may be inactivated by retrotransposons. Retrotransposons are particles of retroviral origin embedded in the human genome. Human DNA consists of 42% retrotransposons, which are partly inactive [6]. In embryogenesis retrotransposons can switch on or off genes by methylation or demethylation or histone acetylation and deacetylation.

Familiar hypo- or hypermelanosis and coat color variegation in mice and dogs are caused by autosomal mosaicism, for example.

Skin Pattern

The Lines of Blaschko and Dermatomes

The lines of Blaschko should not be confused with dermatomes. Blaschko lines form arcs on the chest, S shapes on the abdomen, and V shapes at the posterior midline [5]. They are thought to reflect the pathways of ectodermal development with transverse migration of cells from the midline primitive streak coupled with longitudinal growth and flexion of the embryo [5], which explains the whorly pattern.

Dermatomes correspond to the innervated areas of sensory nerves, which result from the segmental arrangement of the somites. Whether skin lesions follow the Blaschko lines or the dermatomes depends on when the mutation took place.

Segmental Manifestations

Dermatoses with autosomal dominant heredity may manifest as mosaicisms, and two different types can be distinguished: type I and type II segemental manifestation see (Figure 1) [9].

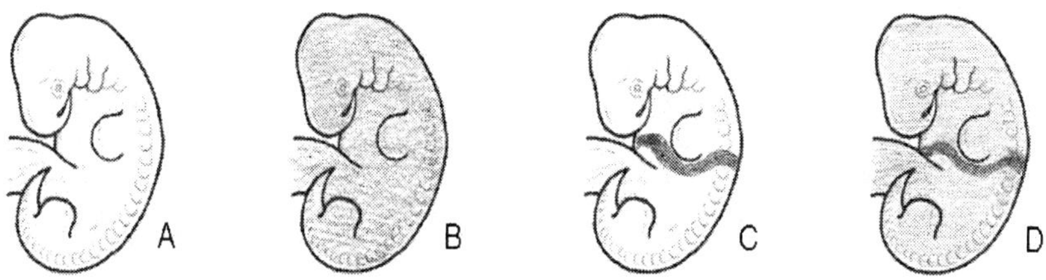

Figure 1 A. unaffected, B: heterozygote, C: Type I segmental, D: Type II segmental.

A. Type I Segmental Manifestation

This type is derived from an early postzygotic mutation in a healthy embryo. The skin lesions are present in Blaschko-linear or other mosaic pattern that correspond to the distribution of cells that exhibit the mutation, and the background skin has normal appearance and genotype [5, 9].

If the mutation affects the patient´s gonads as well, the individual´s offspring could develop the full-blown disorder [5].

Diseases with a possible type I segmental manifestations are neurofibromatosis type I, Darier´s disease and pachyonychia congenital.

B. Type II Segmental Manifestation

A type II segmental manifestation can be seen in autosomal dominant diseases. If the wild type allele is lost in a heterozygous individual by postzygotic recombination, for example, the more severe lesions manifest in one segment, which is superimposed on the diffuse distribution of the other milder skin lesions. A family history of the condition may or may not be known, because the germline heterozygous mutation could have been inherited or could have been arisen de novo. Chances of passing on the general condition to the offspring are approximately 50% [5]. In 2004 this concept was first proven on the molecular level in Hailey-Hailey disease [10]. Other diseases that manifest in a segmental type II pattern are Darier´s disease (Figure 2a and b), cutaneous leiomyomatosis, glomangiomatosis, and disseminated superficial actinic porokeratosis. The mechanism that likely explains the early-onset of squamous cell carcinoma in disseminated superficial actinic porokeratosis due to the loss of heterozygosity can be interpreted as the first step toward carcinogenesis [11].

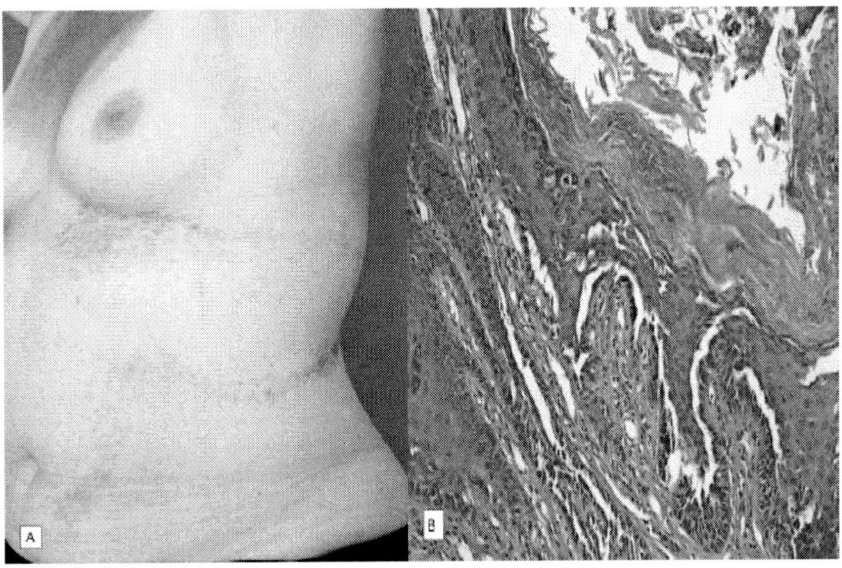

Figure 2A. Clinical presentation: Female patient with a diffuse distribution of Darier´s disease involving the entire body. Additionally, at the trunk manifestation in a blaschko-linear pattern. Figure 2B: Histology of lesional skin reveals focal suprabasal akantholysis with parakeratosis and dyskeratosis, corps ronds and grains.

Patterns of Cutaneous Mosaicism

The pattern of cutaneous mosaicism depends on the type of cell that is affected and its trajectory of migration and proliferation during embryogenesis. Five different patterns have been described by Happle (Figure 3) [4].

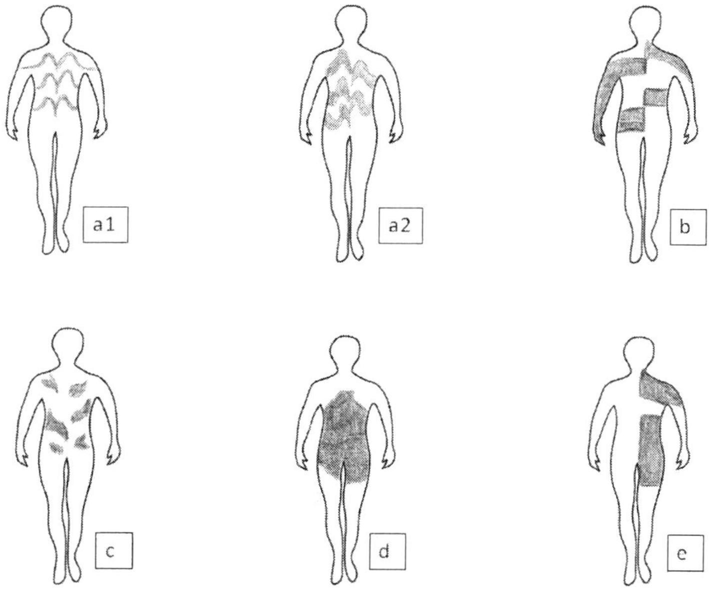

Figure 3. Pattern of cutaneous mosaicism according to Happle a1: Blaschko linear type with narrow bands, a2: Blaschko linear type with broad bands, b: blocklike type, c: phylloid type, d: large patches without midline separation, e: lateralization type.

A. Blaschko Linear Type with Broad or Narrow Bands

Because the course of Blaschko-lines reflects ectodermal development, mostly keratinocytes or melanocytes are involved [12]. The pattern usually presents in classic narrow bands, but broader bands can be observed as well.

Mosaic skin conditions that follow the Blaschko lines

- Incontinentia pigmenti
- Lichen striatus
- Blaschkitis
- Hypomelanosis of Ito
- McCune-Albright syndrome
- Epidermal nevi
- ILVEN
- Porokeratosis linearis unilateralis
- Linear Lupus erythematodes

Incontinentia Pigmenti

Incontinentia pigmenti (IP) is an x-linked dominant disorder, lethal in the majority of male individuals, and variably expressed in females [16]. Four stages of the disease can be distinguished as seen in Table 1:

The gene for incontinentia pigmenti has been mapped to Xp28. Mutations of the NEMO/IKK gene located at Xq28 have been found to cause expression of the disease [16]. Cells that are IKK deficient are likely to undergo apoptosis. Release of cell components then leads to IKK complex activation in keratinocytes without this mutation. Release of TNF-α and IL-1β leads, in turn, to eotaxin enhancement in blood vessel endothelia and to extravasation of eosinophilic granulocytes. The latter migrate into the epidermis and cause the typical histological finding of IP; namely, eosinophilic spongiosis [16].

Table 1.

Stage	Skin lesions
I	Erythema and vesicules in a Blaschko-linear pattern
II	Verrucous and hyperkeratotic papules and plaques
III	Whorly and streaky hyperpigmentations
IV	Pale, bold, atrophic and hypopigmented maculae

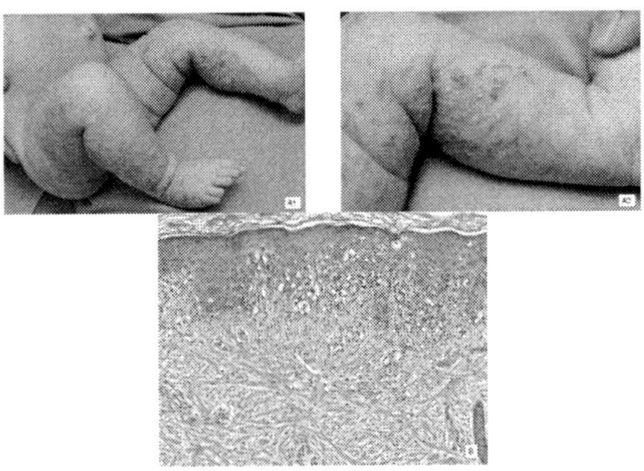

Figure 4A and B. Incontinentia pigmenti in a 2-month old girl, vesicular stage. Figure 4c Histomorphology is presented with typical feature of eosinophilic spongiosis.

Complete apoptosis of all cells with a mutation in NEMO gene indicates the end of stage I and the beginning of stage II of the disease.

However, there is no causative therapy, and it can remain symptomatic only. But patients have to be carefully screened for extracutaneous manifestation, such as dental abnormalities like anodontia or partial absence of teeth (more than 80%), ocular abnormalities like strabismus, crossed eyes or optic nerve atrophy, neurologic impairment like mental retardation or epilepsy, and onychodystrophia [16].

Hypomelanosis of Ito (Incontinentia Pigmenti Achromians)

Hypomelanosis of Ito was first described in 1952 by Minor Ito of Japan. He noticed the skin lesions as a negative of the skin lesions in seen in Incontinentia pigmenti [18]. Individuals show skin hypopigmentations along the Blaschko-lines due to the diminished number of melanocytes in the skin. Although first described as a purely cutaneous disease, various extracutaneous manifestations are now known: epilepsy, mental retardation, skoliosis, strabismus, atrophy of the optical nerve, and dental abnormalities as well as hardness of hearing [19].

Lichen Striatus and Blaschikits – All the Same or Different Entities?

Blaschkitis (BL) and lichen striatus (LS) are rare dermatoses that occur along the Blaschko lines of the skin that exhibit preferential occurrence in distinct age categories [17]. It remains controversial whether these diseases are two different entities or two parts of the wide spectrum of blaschkolinear dermatoses.

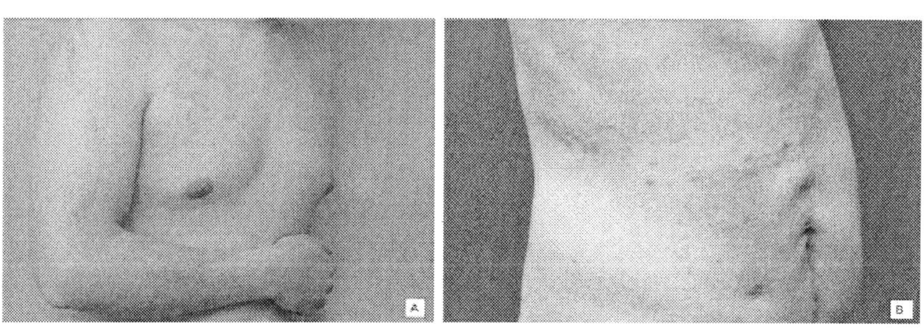

Figure 5. A: Patient with Lichen striatus, B: Patient with Blaschkitis.

Whereas Lichen striatus is more common and occurs mostly in children, Blaschkitis is a rare disease mostly seen in adults (Figure 5a,b). Lichen striatus affects the limbs, Blaschkitis first and foremost the trunk. Resolution of LS is slow whereas Blaschkitis is rapid; relapses in Blaschkitis are more frequent and rarely seen in LS [17].

ILVEN (Inflammatory Linear Verrucous Epidermal Nevus)

Inflammatory linear verrucous epidermal nevus (ILVEN) is an unusual unilateral eruption with onset usually in infancy or childhood, female predominance, frequent left leg involvement, pruritus, refractoriness to therapy, and a psoriasiform histologic pattern (see Figure 6) [20].

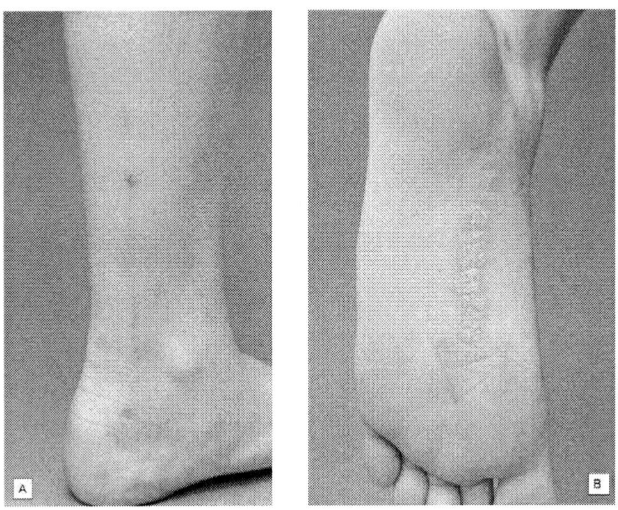

Figure 6. Patient with ILVEN on the left leg.

B. Blocklike (Checkerboard)Type

This type is mostly observed on the trunk, but squares can also occur on the extremities. Some birthmarks described as segmental, dermatomal or zosteriform may also be included in this group [13]. This mosaicism can affect mesodermal derivates such as fibroblasts, blood vessels, neural tissues, and so forth. Café-au-lait macules, speckled lentiginous nevi, or Becker nevi may present in blocklike pattern.

Mosaic skin conditions with blocklike manifestation

- Becker nevus
- Nevus comedonicus
- Café-au-lait spot
- Segmental vitiligo
- Cutis marmorata teleangiectatica congenita
- Plexiform neurofibroma
- Speckled lentiginous nevus

C. Phylloid Type

The best and most common example of a phylloid pattern is phylloid hypomelanosis, which may also be associated with mental retardation, loss of hearing, or skeletal defects. A mosaic partial or complete trisomy 13 has been found in this phenotype and is thought to be related to the 13q region [14].

D. Large Patches without Midline Separation Type

Skin lesions most frequently seen in large patches without midline separation are large congenital nevi which may form a bathing-suit-like pattern.

Mosaic skin conditions that manifest as large patches without midline separation

- large congenital (bathing-suit) nevi
- neurocutaneous melanosis

E. Lateralization Type

The only lateralization type dermatosis that manifests is CHILD syndrome, the congenital hemidysplasia with ichthyosiform nevus and limb defects. It is an x-linked male-lethal disorder caused by a mutation of the NSDHL (NADPH steroid dehydrogenaselike) gene, which encodes an enzyme involved in cholesterol biosynthesis [5].

This pattern has been postulated to reflect the interplay between lionization and a clone of organizer cells that controls a lager morphogenetic field [5, 15].

Epidermal Nevus Syndromes

Skin lesions can also be the first sign of a systemic disease. Several epidermal nevi, which also display a cutaneous mosaicism, may play a decisive role. In addition, it may be the dermatologist who alerts other clinicians to the diagnosis.

Table 2.

Syndrome	Genetics	Skin lesions	Other findings
CHILD syndrome	X-chromosomal dominant	Inflammatory ichthyosiform nevus	Ipsilaterale Hypoplasia of musles or skeleton, reduced thermo- or analgesia, epilepsy, organic heart defects, hypoplasia of kidney or lung
Schimmelpenning-Feuerstein-Mims syndrome	sporadic	Blaschko-linear sebaceus nevus	Mental retardation, epilepsy, coloboma of the iris
Nevus comedonicus syndrome	sporadic	Blaschko-linear nevus comedonicus	Ipsilateral cataract, skeletal malformation, epilepsy
Becker-Nevus syndrome	Paradominant	Pigmented and hairy epidermal nevus on the shoulder	Ipsilateral hypoplasia of M. pectoralis and/or subcutaneous fat or skeleton
Proteus syndrome	sporadic, paradominant	Epidermal nevus, subcutaneous hamartomas, anomaly of blood vessels	Partial gigantism, hemimegaenzephalia, macrodaktylia

Table 2 gives an overview of the various epidermal nevus syndromes with consideration to genetics, skin lesions, and other findings.

The most famous person with an epidermal nevus syndrome is Joseph Merrick (1862-1880); he suffered from a Proteus syndrome. In 1980 David Lynch created a film based on his life called, “The Elephant Man”.

Conclusion

It has been a long journey from the time when Alfred Blaschko first detected the lines now known as Blaschko lines to the final understanding their true meaning and significance. The concept of cutaneous mosaicism has now been proven on the molecular level.

Happle described five patterns of cutaneous mosaicism: Blaschko linear pattern with broad or narrow bands, the checkerboard pattern, the phylloid pattern, the pattern with large patches without midline separation, and the lateralization pattern.

Genomic cutaneous mosaicism and epigenetic mosaicism can be distinguished. Genomic mosaicism can be caused by half-cromatid mutation in a gamete, postzygotic mutation, revertant mosaicism or paradominant inheritance, whereas epigenetic mosaicism is caused by retrotransposons and can affect the x-chromosome or autosomes. Moreover, nevi reflect cutaneous mosaicism and can be the first sign of a systemic disease in epidermal nevus syndromes.

Hence, cutaneous mosaicism plays an important role in the diagnosis of disease and also in furthering the understanding of the underlying genetic mechanisms.

References

[1] Blaschko, A. (1901). Die Nervenverteilung in der Haut in ihrer Beziehung zu den Erkrankungen der Haut. Vienna and Leipzig: Braunmüller.

[2] Jackson, R. (1976). The lines of Blaschko: a review and reconsideration: observations of the cause of certain unusual linear conditions of the skin. *Br J Dermatol*, 95, 349-360.

[3] Happle, R. (1977). Genetische Bedeutung der Blaschkoschen Linien. *Z Hautkr*, *52*, 935-944

[4] Happle, R. (1993). Mosaicism in human skin: Understanding the pattern and mechanism. *Arch Dermatol*, *129*, 1460-70

[5] Molho-Pessach, V. (2011). Blaschko lines and other patterns of cutaneous mosaicism. *Clin Dermatol*, *29*, 205-225

[6] Happle, R. (2004). Muster auf der Haut. *Hautarzt*, *55*, 960-968

[7] Yang, T. P. (1988). Spontaneous reversion of novel Lesch-Nyhan mutation by HPRT gene rearrangement. *Somat Cell Mol Genet*, *14*, 293-303

[8] Happle, R. (1999). Loss of heterozygosity in human skin. *J Am Acad Dermatol*, *41*, 143-161

[9] Happle, R. (2001). Segmentale Typ-2-Manifestation autosomal dominanter Hautkrankheiten: entwicklung eines neuen formal-genetischen Konzeptes. *Hautarzt*, *52*, 283-287.

[10] Poplete Gutiérrez, P. (2004). Type 2 segmental Hailey-Hailey disease originatin from loss of heterozygosity: molecular confirmation of a novel clinicogeneteic concept. *Arch Dermatol Res*, *295*, 327.

[11] Happle, R. (2004). Kutane Mosaike: Muster und molekulare Mechanismen. *Deutsches Ärzteblatt*, *26*, 1886-1891.

[12] Moss, C. (1999). Cytogenetic and molecular evidence for cutaneous mosaicism: the ectoermal origin of Blascko lines. *Am J Med Genet*, *331*, 1408-15.

[13] Torrelo, A. (2005). Delineation of the various shapes and patterns of nevi. *Eur J Dermatol*, *15*, 439-50.

[14] Gonzalez-Ensenat, M. A. (2009). Phylloid hypomelanosis and mosaic partial trisomy 13: two cases that provide further evidence of a distinct clinicogenetic entity. *Arch Dermatol*, *145*, 576-8.

[15] Happle, R. (2006). X-chromosome inactivation: role in skin disease expression. *Acta Paediatr*, *95*, 16-23.

[16] Berlin, AL. (2002). Incontinentia pigmenti: a review and an update on the molecular basis of pathophysiology. *J Am Acad Dermatol*, *47*, 169-87.

[17] Müller, CSL. (2010). Lichen striatus and blaschkitis – reappraisal of the concept of blaschkolinear dermatoses, *Br J Dermatol*, *164*, 257-64.

[18] Ito, M. (1952). Studies on melanin XI. Incontinentia pigmenti achromians. A singular case of nevus depigmentosus systemicus bilateralis. *Tohoku J Exp Med*, *55*, 57-59.

[19] Ruggeri, M. (2000). Hypomelanosis of Ito: clinical syndrome or just a phenotype. *J Child Neurol*, *15*(10), 635-44.

[20] Miteva, LG. (2001). Inflammatory linear verrucous epidermal nevus. *Cutis*, *68*(5), 327-30.

In: Dermatitis
Editor: Cornelia Sigrid Lissi Müller
ISBN: 978-1-62618-997-3

Chapter V

Borreliosis (Lyme Disease)

***Klaus Eisendle*[1,*], *Jenny Deluca*[1] *and Bernhard Zelger*[2]**
[1]Department of Dermatology Central Teaching Hospital
Bolzano/Bozen, Italy
[2]Department of Dermatology, Innsbruck Medical University,
Innsbruck, Austria

Abstract

Borreliosis (Lyme disease) is the most common zoonosis in the northern hemisphere. The pathogen, a spirochetal bacterium, *Borrelia burgdorferi* is transmitted by ticks of the *Ixodes ricinus* species complex. Borreliosis has a variety of presentations at different stages of infection and often leads to various skin affections, but might also compromise multiple organs, especially the central and peripheral nervous system, joints and muscles. Although Lyme disease is known for almost 20 years the known spectrum of its skin manifestations is continuously expanding and cannot be regarded as completed. Besides the classical manifestations of cutaneous borreliosis like erythema (chronicum) migrans, borrelial lymphocytoma and acrodermatitis chronica atrophicans evidence is growing that in part also other skin manifestations, especially morphea, lichen sclerosus and cases of cutaneous B-cell lymphoma are causally related to infections with Borrelia. Also cutaneous sarcoidosis, granuloma annulare and interstitial granulomatous dermatitis might be partly caused

* Correspondence: Klaus.eisendle@asbz.it.

by Borrelia burgdorferi or similar strains. There are also single reports of other skin manifestations to be associated with borrelial infections like necrobiosis lipoidica and necrobiotic xanthogranuloma. In addition, as the modern chameleon of dermatology, cutaneous borreliosis, especially borrelial lymphocytoma, mimics other skin conditions, as has been shown for erythema annulare centrifugum or lymphocytic infiltration of the skin (Jessner Kanof).

Definition

Lyme disease is currently the most common arthropod-born infectious disease in temperate regions of the northern hemisphere. It is a multisystemic inflammatory disorder caused by the slowly growing microaerophil gram negative spirochetes belonging to the *Borrelia burgdorferi-sensu-lato* complex.

Lyme borreliosis is transmitted from animals to humans by hard-bodied ticks (Ixodes). Those ticks are generalists, feeding on a multitude of vertebrates such as mice, shrews, deer and birds [1-6].

History

Although in 1978 Allen Steere provided the first description of arthritis with cutaneous annular lesion appearing after a thick bite, the cause of the disease remained a mystery until 1981, when a gram negative spirochete, *Borrelia burgdorferi*, was identified in the midgut of the *Ixodes* tick by Willy Burgdorfer.

The denomination of the disease as “Lyme borreliosis” originated in 1986, coming from the town of Lyme (Connecticut), in which the disease occurred more frequently in the 70s of the last century of the last millennium [3-6].

Epidemiology

Lyme Borreliosis emerge focally clustered in the temperate regions of the north hemisphere, with prevalence between 5° E and 25° E longitude and a peak incidence between May and September. The European regions with highest infection rates are Austria, Czech Republic, Germany, Switzerland,

Slovenia and Slovakia. In the USA the most endemic regions are the north-eastern and north-central states.

Due to the lack of mandatory reports of cases of borreliosis, the precise incidence of this disease is not known. The estimated incidence of borreliosis in central Europe has been growing since the 1980s and now ranges from 50 - >400 cases per 100,000 persons per year. Seroprevalence in children and adolescence is 5% throughout Germany, suggesting an early contact with the pathogen and reaches as high values as 30% in healthy adult blood donors from highly endemic areas of Austria.

The rate of infected ticks in endemic regions is very variable; data coming from a recent metaanalysis show an overall mean prevalence of Borrelia in ticks of 13.7%, but higher values up to 60% have been reported. Approximately every tenth tick bite in endemic areas has a Borrelia infection as result. Both sexes and all age groups may be affected [7-9].

Ecology and Disease Transmission

The Gram-negative B. burgdorferi has a spiral structure with a width of 0.2μm to 0.3 μm and a length ranging from 20 μm to 30 μm. This bacterium is comprised of a trilaminar outer membrane surrounding a protoplasmic cylinder. It has about 7-12 periplasmic endoflagella, which are responsible for its structural morphology and motility.

B. burgdorferi was the first spirochete for which the complete genome was sequenced. It consists in a small sized linear chromosome of about 1000 kilobases, also present are 21 plasmid (12 circular and 9 linear). It does not contain any genes involved in biosynthetic pathways, making the microorganism dependent on its environment for nutritional requirements. This explains why the growth and the various geographical distribution of B. burgdorferi depend on the availability of competent animals in the area.

Currently, the B. burgdorferii sensu lato (sl) complex comprises at least 18 genospecies. They show different geographic distribution, for example, B. garinii and B. afzelii are frequently found in Europe, followed by B. burdorferii sensu strictu (ss) and B. valaisana, while B. burgdorferii ss is the most common type in USA.

Differences within the bacterial strains explain the different patterns of pathogenicity and tissue tropism. Indeed B. burgdorferi ss affects frequently the joints, B. garinii shows a preference for the nervous system, while B.

afzelii is mostly associated with skin manifestation. Species like B. bisettii, B. japonica or B. californiensis do not seem to affect humans.

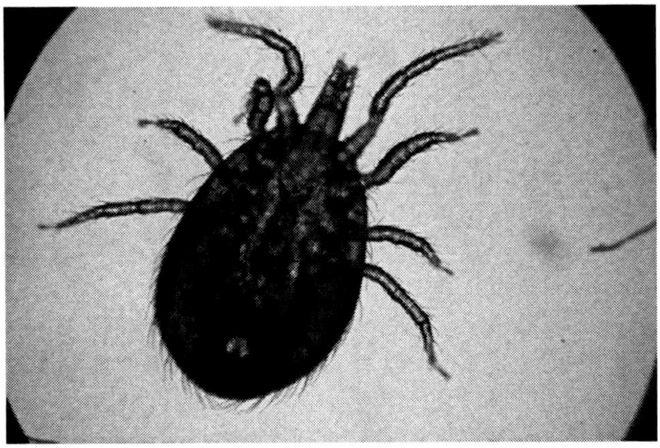

Figure 1. Ixodes ricinus tick.

The principal vector of B. burgdorferi infection is the Ixodes (I.) tick. In Europe it is I. ricinus (Figure 1.), while in Asia is I. persulcatum and in USA I. scapularis or I. pacificus.

These ticks have 2-year life cycle with three successive, seasonal life stages. Adult female ticks lay eggs which hatch and become larvae, subsequently nymph, and then adult.

A single blood meal is taken in each stage. Ticks acquire the Borrelia-spirochete bacterium by feeding on an infected host or when feeding very close to an infected tick, or by feeding from the site where another infected tick has recently bitten.

Necessary hosts for immature stages in the life cycle of the tick, and therefore the main reservoirs for those spirochetes, are small vertebrate such as rodents, insectivores, hares and several bird species, while adult ticks may infest larger mammals, especially deer.

Ticks dwell primarily on the underside of plant up to about 1 m above the ground. They perceive a potential host through the use of chemoreceptors. After contact with the animal they search out warm areas of the body with very thin skin and then start to bite.

During the passage from an invertebrate to a vertebrate the spirochete encounters two different environments. On one hand the different immune systems: the innate immune system of the tick and then the well-developed adaptive immune systems of mammals and birds. On the other hand the temperature: from the range of ambiental temperature (ticks do not thermoregulate) to a constant mammalian's temperature. To ensure its survival the genome of Borrelia contains several plasmid-encoded surface lipoproteins, indeed, in place of a typical lipopolysaccharide coat, these spirochetes have multiple antigenic surface lipoproteins. These include outer surface proteins (Osp) A and F, a variable surface antigen (VlsE), a fibronectin-binding protein (BBK32), and decorin-binding proteins (DbpA and DbpB), which expression is upregulated or downregulated depending on its life cycle. Indeed Borrelia remains unarmed in an infected tick until it feeds. The dormant spirochete must express surface lipoproteins OspA and B, which function as adhesion molecules, in order to colonize the tick midgut. When the ticks feed, alterations in temperature and pH in the midgut activate the bacteria to undergo phenotypic changes, namely OspA is downregulated, and the surface proteins OspC and DbpA are upregulated, which allows its translocation in the host tick's salivary glands. The injection of infected saliva during a prolonged feeding period (usually > 17 hours are needed) promotes the transmission of B. burgdorferii by I. ricinus. After the tick bite, Borrelia disseminate from the inoculation site through blood or other body tissues.

In Europe ticks of the species Ixodes ricinus can also transmit other pathogens (co-infection), which may confuse the clinical findings of Lyme disease. It is the case of the flavivirus causing the tick-borne encephalitis (TBE), the obligate intracellular gram-negative bacteria Anaplasma phagocyphilum, causative agent of the human granulocytic anaplasmosis, Bartonella spp. and the protozoon Babesia, responsible for a malaria-like disease with fever, anemia and jaundice [7, 10-14].

Clinical Manifestations

Signs and symptoms of Lyme disease, similar to syphilis, are often divided into stages with also asymptomatic periods. This arbitrary division is actually didactically useful and sometimes not in agreement with clinical findings. Many of the manifestations of this disease are caused by active infection by the spirochete; others may be driven by immunopathogenetic mechanisms. Moreover the clinical findings depend also from the genospecies of Borrelia, immunity of the host and several other predisposing factors [1-5].

Clinical Manifestations of Cutaneous Borreliosis

1. Early Localized Disease

The first skin manifestation usually occurs 1 to 3 weeks after the infection and is recognized in approximately 75–90% of patients with objective evidence of Lyme borreliosis. It is characterized at the site of inoculation by *erythema migrans* (EM), an eruption that begins as an erythematous macule or papule, usually in a ring formation, that spreads centrifugally and rapidly (Figure 2.).

It may develop a central clearing producing a target-like morphology. The size of erythema may vary in general from 10 to 20 cm in diameter. The minimum diameter is usually about 5 cm, while in individual cases were observed lesions even reaching >70 cm in diameter. The development of multiple EM lesions in a single patient is also possible.

In principle all body areas may be affected, with the exception of palmar-plantar zones, but generally EM is most seen in particular regions: e.g the armpit-shoulder area, the thigh-groin, buttock region, or calf-popliteal fossa region in adults; head and neck regions in children. EM develops due to local spread of the spirochetes; about half of patients report only a slight itching or burning localized to the inoculation site as associated symptoms.

The initial skin infection is not always clinically typical. *Borrelia*s are also detected in homogeneous reddish and non-migrating erythemas, as well as patchy infiltrated erythemas, erysipeloid flaming red erythemas and in erythemas with vesiculation.

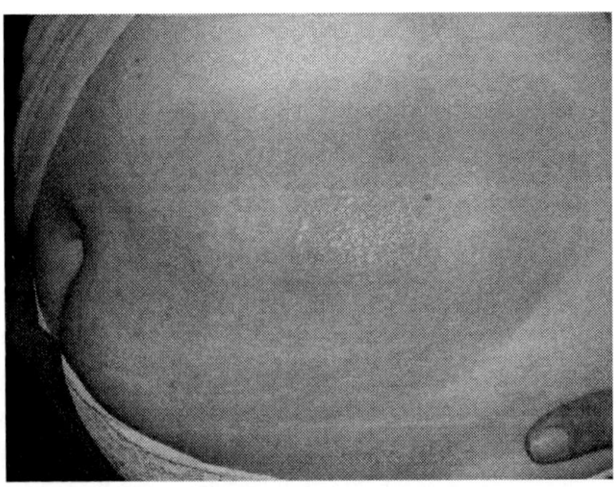

Figure 2. Erythema migrans.

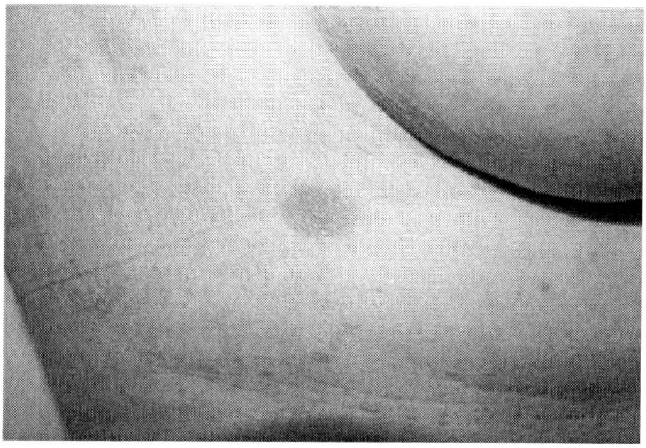

Figure 3. Borrelial lymphocytoma.

Borrelial lymphocytoma (BL), also named lymphadenosis benigna cutis, is a B-cell-"pseudolymphoma" that represents an immunologic reaction to the presence of *B. burgdorferi* as antigenic stimulus in the skin. It commonly appears like an indolent, soft, sharply demarcated bluish-red papular-nodular-tumoral lesion, usually 0.5-5 cm large (Figure 3.). It is often solitary and observed more often in children than in adults. It is frequently located on the ear lobes, scrotum in children and near nipple areola in adults. Unusual localization may be external genitalia or the anterior axillary fold. Coexistence with EM is possible. The BL can persist from months to years. After a first rapid response to an antibiotic therapy it takes usually weeks to months to completely disappear.

Complicated clinical courses are at this time generally avoided by adequate therapy. Without treatment the infection can proceed and disseminate with multiorgan involvement [1-5, 15-18].

2. Early Disseminated Disease

A hematogenous dissemination is possible already in the early stage in about one to two thirds of patients. This is clinical recognizable due to the occurrence of extra-cutaneous symptoms. They are generally unspecific, mild and short lived, comprising flu-like symptoms, e.g. fatigue, fever, headache, chills, vertigo, nausea, anorexia, beside regional lymphadenopathy. Single to multiple EMs or late borrelial lymphocytomas are visible in this stage. Multiple EMs often present with ovoid shape, well-defined edges and without epidermal involvement. In the case of absent or atypical EM this stage is more difficult to recognize [15-18].

3. Chronic Disease with Organ Involvement

The dissemination occurs in a wide range of time, varying from one week to one month after the primary infection. The involvement of the musculoskeletal system occurs with acute arthritis, painful muscles, tendons, bursae and bones. Common signs of a nervous implication are meningitis, lymphocytic meningoradiculoneuritis (Bannwarth syndrome), mild encephalitis and myelitis. Possible manifestations of heart involvement are atrioventricular block, myopericarditis and pancarditis. In the last stage of the disease it is possible to observe damage in joints, nervous system or skin, which may be functional or irreversible [5].

Skin Manifestations of the Late Stage

The dermatological stigma of this stage is acrodermatitis chronica atrophicans (ACA) (Figure 4.). It is mostly associated with B. afzelii infection, which explains why this condition is almost exclusively found in Europe. It occurs months to years after the initial tick bite and begins with an inflammatory phase. ACA has been observed mainly in ederly patients, particulary women. Commonly the affected patients were bitten repeatedly for years or are outdoor workers in endemic areas, although almost no one is able to recall a tick bite. ACA begins with an inflammatory phase: edematous cutaneous papules to patches and plaques with bluish-red discoloration are detectable on the extensor surfaces of fingers, hands, joints and lower extremities. The infiltrative process may affect also the face and be confused with lupus erythematodes. Those first inflammatory manifestations do not resolve spontaneously, in the absence of treatment the lesions progress over many weeks to months into an atrophic phase. The skin loses gradually the epidermal and dermal structures, becoming thin, wrinkled („cigarette paper-like“ skin atrophy) and, in advanced cases, hyperpigmented, dry, hairless, with multiple teleangiectases and prominence of superficial veins. In a subset of ACA patients (10-20%), due to a focally increased production of dermal collagen, there are visible indurated bands most often along the ulna or tibia and/or fibrotic nodules of the dorsal aspects of the elbows.

The most frequent extracutaneous manifestation of ACA is peripheral neuropathy (muscular weakness, dysaesthesias, pain and muscle cramps), in patients with long-standing disease abnormalities in bones and joints (subluxation or luxations, bursitis, arthritis, periosteal bone thickening) are also present [4, 15-18].

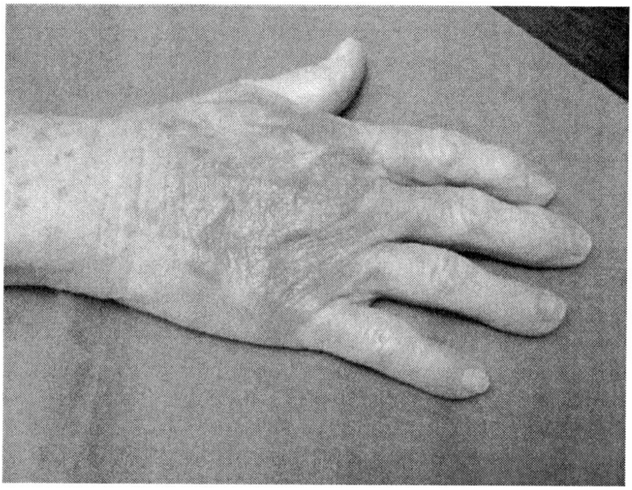

Figure 4. Acrodermatitis chronica atrophicans.

New Emerging "Lyme-Like" Diseases

During the past two decades, physicians working in nonendemic regions of the USA, e.g. Southeast and South Central United States reported an illness characterized by the presence of expanding annular erythema migrans-like rash and mild flu-like symptoms following a history of tick bite. This Lyme disease mimic is now being recognized as a separate disease, precisely as southern tick–associated rash illness (STARI) or Masters disease. STARI does not appear to be caused by *Borrelia burgdorferi sensu stricto*. The exact etiology is still uncertain, the probable bacterial cause of this Lyme like Borreliosis is an uncultivable borrelia, known as *Borrelia lonestari,* found in the Lone Star ticks *(Amblyomma americanum),* named after the prominent white dot on the back of the adult female. At presence, there is no serologic antibody test available to detect *B. lonestari* and the diagnosis is based on a suggestive clinic. Symptoms resolve quickly after antibiotic treatment.

A similar condition has been reported in brazilian patients, who, after a tick bite episode, developed symptoms as erythema migrans, general flu-like symptoms and arthritis. The Brazilian zoonosis was named Baggio-Yoshinari Syndrome (BYS). Ticks not belonging to the *Ixodes ricinus* complex have been detected as vectors, whereas the causal agents seem to be latent spirochetes with atypical (cystic) morphology. Also in the case of BYS the diagnosis is essentially clinical.

In our opinion, it seems likely that this newer described forms of EM are caused by different yet to be better characterized endemic Borrelial strains as it is the case in Europe by *B. burgdorferi ss*, *B. garinii* and *B. afzelii* [19-23].

Borrelia Burgdorferi and "Non Classical" Skin Diseases

The classical spectrum of skin manifestations in Lyme disease has been gradually expanding. There is now growing evidence that other skin diseases like morphea, lichen sclerosus and cases of primary cutaneous B-cell lymphoma (PCBCL) are in part caused by infections with *Borrelia sp.*.

The pathogenetic links between PCBCL and *B. burgdorferi* infection comes from parallels with *Helicobacter pylorii* infection and MALT lymphomas. A prolonged *Borrelia* infection may cause a chronic lymphatic stimulation which subsequently leads to developing slowly growing, poorly defined erythematous nodules and tumors on the skin. In European studies there is evidence of a positive association between Lyme borreliosis, in particular the strain *B. afzelii*, and malignant cutaneous lymphomas. That demonstration has failed in North America and Asia. Differences in *B. burgdorferi* strains between different endemic regions may provide the explanation; *B. afzelii* appears to be the predominant strain in Europe, while *B. burgdorferi sensu stricto* is more common in North America.

The involvement of *B. burgdorferi sl.* as causative agent of circumscribed scleroderma (morphea), an inflammatory connective tissue disease, was firstly proposed by Aberer et al in 1985 [24]. Different studies could confirm the presence of Borrelia in patients with morphea using serological, immuno-histochemical, culture and PCR approaches.

Some patients with morphea show clinical similarities to classical borreliosis. Early stages of morphea with prominent lilac ring are even sometimes difficult to distinguish from EM with its active border, whereas in late stages red-purple-brown macules of burned out morphea may mimic ACA (Figure 5.). There are also similarities in the histopathological findings between EM, ACA and morphea. They include: variable infiltrate of lymphocytes, macrophages and plasma cells; slight vacuolar degeneration of the basal layer in the late stages; an increase of fibrocytes/fibroblasts with variable fibrosis to sclerosis. A bacterial etiology is further suggested because some cases of morphea respond well to antibiotic therapy, such as penicillin and ceftriaxone. D-penicillamine, discussed in older text books as inhibiting cross connection between collagen fibers, was likely to have been effective because of its metal-chelating activity which deprived the bacterial of essential trace elements such as manganese, zinc and magnesium. The collagenotropism of *Borrelia* is further supported by the presence of fibronectin binding proteins which promote bacterial attachment to glycosaminoglicans of the connective tissue between collagen bundles. Nevertheless, the low level of microorganisms found in the lesions probably indicates that the disease is not only due to the effect of the infective agent, but also reflects the challenge for the immune system due to the location of the spirochete and or even a compromised immune reaction in morphea patients themselves, where *Borrelia* might trigger a subsequent autoimmune reaction.

Figure 5. Morphea.

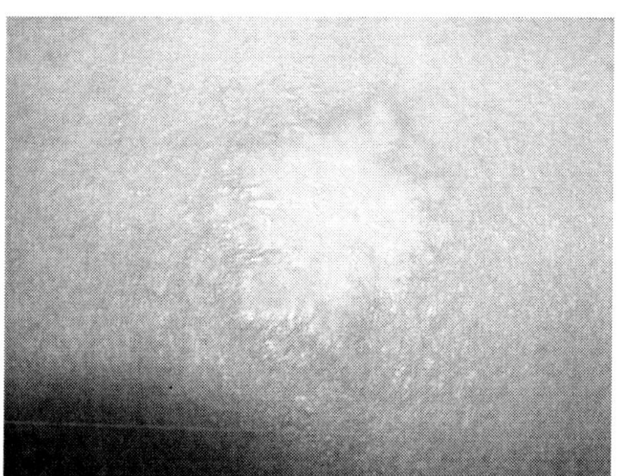

Figure 6. Lichen sclerosus et atrophicus of the dorsal skin.

Another cutaneous disease that shares clinical and histological similarities with morphea is lichen sclerosus (LS). LS, in literature reported also as lichen sclerosus et atrophicus, is a chronic inflammatory skin disease of unknown etiology mainly affecting the anogenital skin of females but also of males and the general skin. The lesions appear whitish, sharply demarcated, with solitary papules to converging plaques. The surface of the lesions may be elevated or in the same plane as normal skin, whereas in advanced stages they may be depressed (Figure 6). LS shares similarities and common features with ACA, including histological findings such as infiltrate of lymphocytes admixed with some plasma cells, an increase of fibrocytes and fibroblasts and diffuse dermal fibrosis to sclerosis. These observations have led several investigators to consider the possibility of *B. burgdorferi* as common etiologic factor for both diseases. The infectious hypothesis with spirochetes helps to explain the most common stereotypical presentation of LS, namely in the genitoanal area. Indeed, in early borrelial infection a subclinical dissemination of the spirochetes to kidney and urine frequently occurs. Subsequently the moist and traumatisms of genitalia allow the spirochetes to reinfect the superficial tissues of the perigenital region. This also explains why other mucous membranes, such as the oral or endonasal mucosa and conjunctiva, compared to the perigenital region are practically never affected.

In the literature, besides primary cutaneous B-cell lymphoma, morphea and LS, other especially granulomatous skin diseases are described as known and possible skin manifestations in cutaneous borreliosis. Indeed evidence is growing that granuloma annulare and interstitial granulomatous dermatitis might be partly caused by *B. burgdorferi* or similar strains. Also cases of cutaneous sarcoidosis have been linked to Borrelia, especially in the Chinese literature. It is not unlikely that chronic presence of borrelial spirochetes in the skin – in analogy to *Treponema pallidum* in tertiary syphilis and as seen in other chronic skin infections, such as cutaneous (atypical) tuberculosis, lepra or leishmaniosis – lead to formation of granulomas.

There are single reports which connect other skin disease to *Borrelia*, for example necrobiosis lipoidica, necrobiotic xanthogranuloma and single cases of mycosis fungoides, but the evidence for latter skin disease are not unambiguous. In addition, as the modern chameleon of dermatology, cutaneous borreliosis, especially BL, mimics other skin conditions, as has been shown for erythema annulare centrifugum or lymphocytic infiltration of the skin (Jessner-Kanof). For an overview of skin manifestations associated with borrelial infections see Figure 7 [24-33].

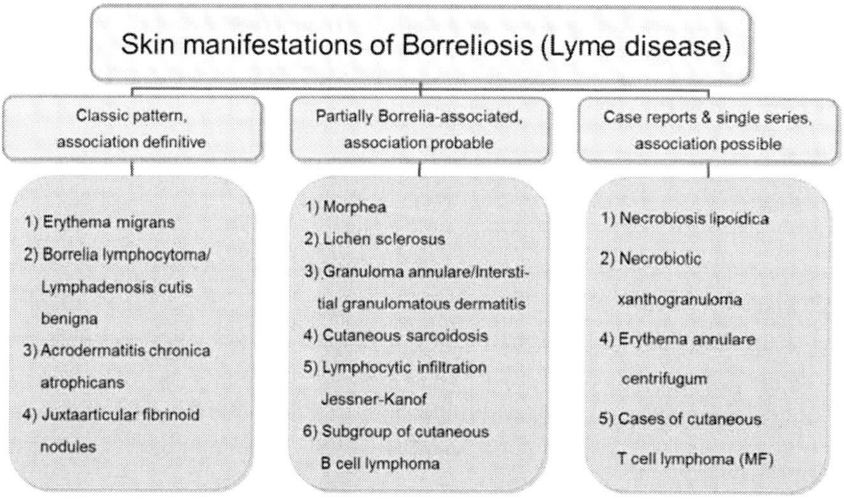

Figure 7. Skin manifestations associated with cutaneous borreliosis as reported in the literature.

Histopathologic Patterns in Classical Cutaneous Borreliosis

The dermopathological changes in cutaneous borreliosis are a consequence of the continuous antigenic stimulus by persisting *Borrelia* in the tissue. The consequences are histopathologic similarities in between the different cutaneous manifestations, like structural changes in the collagen texture and the frequent presence of B lymphocytes, especially plasma cells.

The different clinical and histological manifestation can be explained by the localization and duration of the infection and by the different known borrelial strains, on the other hand also by the dominating immune response involving B and T cells, as well as the number of inoculated bacteria and the genetic predisposition of the infected host. The damage in the connective tissue collagen is on one hand the result of the inflammatory infiltrate ("cytokine storm", collateral damage), on the other hand *Borrelia* show collagentropism and might directly influence and damage the collagen structure. Histopathology of classical cutaneous borrelioses is characteristic, but unfortunately not very specific, meaning that the diagnosis is first of all mainly a clinical one.

In the case of EM histopathology shows perivascular lymphocytic infiltrations not always containing plasma cells in all the dermal layers, sometimes with admixture of eosinophilic granulocytes and macrophages, as well as slight changes in the structure of collagen texture in the connective tissue.

Some authors consider BL as special form of an EM. Histopathology shows an unremarkable epidermis with sharp defined partially confluent lymphocytic infiltrates. There are two histopathologic types of BL with (follicular type) or without (diffuse/nodular type) follicular structures resembling the germinal centers of lymph nodes. Combination between the two types can be observed. Plasma cells and sometimes eosinophils and multinucleate giant cells can additionally be found at the border of the infiltrate. An unaltered grenz zone between the epidermis and the lymphocytic infiltrate can regularly be observed.

In the cases of ACA depending on the duration of the disease, the changes include more or less pronounced atrophy of the epidermis, dermis and subcutaneous tissue with ectatic capillaries in the upper corium. The inflammatory infiltrate is accentuated perivascular or even band-like and usually contains plasma cells. In addition there is a loss of elastic fibers with the development of fibrosis or incipient sclerosis of the papillary and reticular dermis [15, 35, 36].

Diagnosis

The presence of the typical constellation of signs and symptoms beside the history of a tick bite in a patient living in an endemic area facilitates the clinician to establish the diagnosis of Lyme disease. More difficulties are present for physicians working in nonendemic areas. In those cases it is very important to elicit an accurate anamnesis, including details about prior travels in endemic areas and clinical findings that might be consistent with manifestations of Lyme disease.

The most important clinical finding for diagnosis of early Lyme disease is the characteristic EM lesion. Unfortunately, not all the cases of EM show classical features and it can be misdiagnosed, as either an insect bite or as infection with pyogenic bacteria, and consequently inadequately treated [30, 37].

Direct Identification of the Pathogen

Theoretically the direct cultivation of the B. burgdorferi is the gold standard for the diagnosis of infection, but practically, due to the need of special media (*e.g.* Pettenkofer-Kelly or Barbour-Stoenner-Kelly) and the slow growth and low sensitivity culture is limited to specific laboratories with considerable experience.

In the first microscopic studies *Borrelia* spirochetes were detected using Warthin-Starry silver stain, which allowed displaying just few microorganisms. The histopathologic diagnosis was recently improved by the direct detection of multiple spirochetes by immunohistochemistry and focus floating microscopy (FFM). This technique combines the use of a polyclonal anti-borrelial antibody, which recognizes all different *Borrelial* strains, and a holoscopic approach to the slide by tuning the focus of the microscope through the thickness of the slide (3-4μm). So, with FFM the section is scanned through in two planes: horizontally in serpentines as in routine cytology and simultaneously vertically at magnification of 200 to 400 times. In addition, omission of counterstain and bright illumination of the scanning field (10 times the intensity usually used for routine histologic examination) proved to be very helpful because the bright red 3-amino-9-ethylcarbazole-stained microorganisms best contrasted with the faint yellow of unstained collagen bundles and other tissue structures. FFM is a highly sensitive, reliable, rapid, and inexpensive method to detect and/or confirm *Borrelia* in human tissue (Figure 8) and also in ticks (Figure 9). It works on routinely formalin-fixed, paraffin-embedded tissue samples. Actually, its use is almost confined to academic centers but it is slowly entering as routine in other laboratories [9, 38].

Indirect Detection of the Pathogen

Serologic testing for antibodies to *B. burgdorferi* is often performed in early disease to reinforce the diagnosis but it remains necessary recognizing its limits, above all in this stage. Indeed IgM antibodies against *B. burgdorferi* typically appear within one to two weeks and IgG antibodies usually appear within two to six weeks following the onset of EM. The gap between first skin lesion and the development of a diagnostic, adaptive immune response explains not only the seronegativity in such patients but also its futility as a screening test of asymptomatic patients living in endemic areas or for patients with non-specific symptoms only (e.g., fatigue, myalgias/arthralgias).

Serologic tests became usually positive for both IgM and IgG antibodies to *B. burgdorferi* in early disseminated and late Lyme disease. The performance of a serologic test is therefore adequate in patients with consistent systemic symptoms (e.g. meningitis, radiculopathy, mononeuritis, cranial nerve palsy, arthritis, carditis) and a recent history of having lived or traveled to an area endemic for Lyme disease or history of tick bite exposure. In the case of seronegativity in patients suspected for early disseminated Lyme disease a second serologic testing two weeks after the first assessment is suggested.

Figure 8. Detection of Borrelial spirochetes using Focus Floating Microscopy (400x).

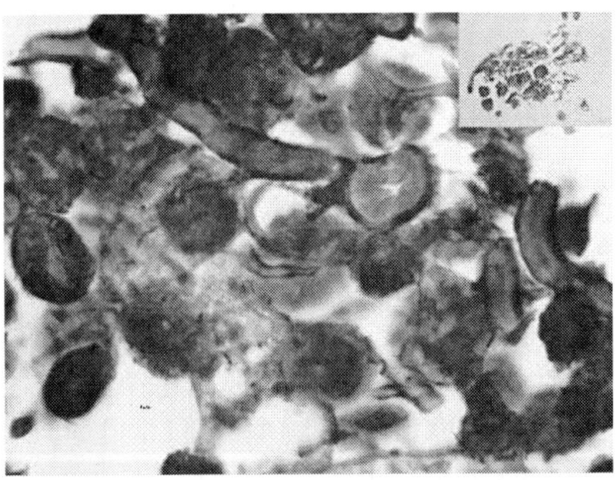

Figure 9. Detection of Borrelial spirochetes in a tick´s (I. ricinus) midgut by FFM (overview 4x, 400x).

Recent recommendations for serologic testing for anti-*B. burgdorferi* antibodies suggest proceeding using a two-tiered system. Either enzyme linked immunosorbent assay (ELISA) or, alternatively, indirect fluorescent antibody test (IFA) are suggested as initial serologic test for supporting the diagnosis of Lyme disease. ELISA detects both IgM and IgG antibody. Considering the possibility of false positive results (e.g. other spirochetal disease, autoimmune disorders) and cross reactions with antibodies synthetized due to nonspecific activation of immunoglobulin production (e.g. EBV, malaria), equivocal or positive results should be followed by a Western blot test. If the ELISA is negative, the sample needs no further testing. In comparison to ELISA the Western blot (or immunoblot) is generally more sensitive and provides more information regarding which antigens of *B. burgdorferi* are reacting with serum antibodies. In the case of a positive ELISA with negative Western blot the results should be considered negative, whereas a positive immunoblot test confirms the contact with *B. burgdorferi*. In Europe, due to the heterogeneity of *Borrelia* strains, the sensitivity of the test may vary depending on the antigen used within the blot. The VlsE C6 epitope is relatively stable between European and US species, and thus VlsE C6 ELISAs may become a more appropriate test for detecting all species of *B. burgdorferi*.

Another diagnostic option is the **polymerase chain reaction (PCR)**. PCR has been used to identify the presence of *B. burgdorferi sensu lato* in different tissues such as skin, CSF, blood and synovial fluid. High specificity rates are reported and evidence indicated that PCR is more accurate than culture and serologic testing in early Lyme disease. However, there are important considerations about the use of this technique, e.g. many different and non-standardized protocols, low sensitivity, its highly technique-dependence and its inability to differentiate between infection with a living bacterial and the presence of remnant DNA from previous, even treated, infection [37, 39-44].

Treatment of Lyme Disease

Actually there is no European consensus on guidelines for Lyme disease treatment. However, on the European Union Concerted Action on Lyme Borreliosis (EUCALB) website are summarized updated treatment regimes and recommendations from European studies. All cases with clinical symptoms should be treated preventing progression to later stages. This also applies to pregnant woman to decrease the risk of adverse outcomes (e.g.

spontaneous abortion, stillbirth, and preterm birth). The type of antibiotic treatment must be adequate for the clinical manifestation [45-49].

Early Disease (Erythema Migrans)

In patients with early disease the efficacies of different therapeutic options have been investigated. The results of the clinical trials converge considering equivalent the efficacy of oral doxycycline, amoxicillin, and cefuroxime axetil for the treatment of early Lyme disease (see Table 1).

Doxycycline is preferred in patients with Lyme disease in endemic areas because it is effective in treating a potential co-infection and shows better penetration into the central nervous system.

Table 1.

Clinical manifestation	Length of therapy	Therapy options
Erythema migrans and Borrelial lymphocytoma	14-21 days	Oral: • Doxycycline 100mg x2/die • Amoxicillin 500mg x3/die • Cefuroxime axetil 500 mg/die
Acrodermatitis chronica atrophicans	21 days	
Neurologic involvement	14 days	Ceftriaxone 2g i.v/die Penicillin G i.v 20 million U/die
	21 days	Doxycycline 100 mg x2/die, oral
Lyme arthritis	28 days	Oral: • Doxycycline 100mg x2/die • Amoxicillin 500-1000 mg x3/die
	21-28 days	Ceftriaxone 2g i.v/die
Cardiac alterations	21 days	Oral: • Doxycycline 100mg x2/die • Amoxicillin 500-1000 mg x3/die or Ceftriaxone 2g i.v/die

Other antibiotic classes, particularly macrolides and first-generation cephalosporins (e.g. cephalexin) should not be used as therapy for erythema migrans because of lower efficacy. The sole exception is azithromycin, which can be an alternative treatment in patients intolerant to antibiotics of first choice or for children and pregnant or breast-feeding women. The treatment duration in most of the above mentioned trials of therapy for erythema migrans were pointed on 21 days. Some studies with doxycycline indicated that shorter treatment regimens (from 10 to 14 days of therapy) might be as effective as more prolonged therapy. A clinical worsening during the first day of therapy is referable to the host immune response to antigens released by dying bacteria, also named Jarisch-Herxheimer reaction [45, 46].

Early Disseminated Disease

The patient's symptoms in the stage of early-disseminated Lyme disease are the mirror of a systemic involvement. In the case of acute neurologic manifestations (e.g. meningitis, cranial neuropathy, and sensory or motor radiculoneuropathy), data coming from different studies performed in Europe suggest treating adults with oral Doxycycline or intravenously therapy with ceftriaxone or penicillin G. Oral doxycycline, whose bioavailability is equivalent to intravenous dosing, is also an alternative drug for patients intolerant of beta-lactam antibiotics and for patients without venous access. Moreover, oral doxycycline is considered the treatment of choice in case of isolated facial nerve palsy [45-46].

Late Disease

Intermittent or chronic Lyme arthritis and cardioborreliosis can usually be treated successfully with oral doxycycline or amoxicillin respectively for four and three weeks. Patients with persistent symptoms may also be treated with intravenous therapy with ceftriaxone. Patients with synovitis may benefit from antiinflammatory therapy or arthroscopic synovectomy. Patients with cardiac manifestations (e.g. atrioventricular block and myopericarditis), beside the antibiotic therapy, should be hospitalized and monitored with cardiac telemetry recurring to a temporary pacemaker in the case of AV block.

Patients with both Lyme arthritis and neurologic manifestations or late neurologic findings should be treated according to the recommendations for early neurologic disease. Acrodermatitis chronica atrophicans should be treated with the same oral regimens that are used for erythema migrans for 3 weeks. See table 1 [45-46].

Post-Treatment Lyme Disease Syndrome

Usually signs and symptoms disappear after antimicrobial therapy. However, a subset of patients treated for Lyme disease report persistent or recurrent symptoms, e.g. fatigue, headache, neurocognitive symptoms, myalgias and arthralgias. The term post-treatment Lyme disease syndrome (PTLDS) was coined to capture the pattern symptoms when they persist for longer than 6 months post-treatment.

The etiology of PTLDS is currently unknown and the hypothesis that in these cases a prolonged antibiotic treatment is needed is a matter of considerable debate. On the one side, there are studies that have assessed the posttreatment persistence of *B. burgdorferi* in animals, e.g. nonhuman primates and rats. Moreover, *B. burgdorferi* have been detected intracellularly in different human cells (endothelium, fibroblasts, synovial cells and neuronal cells) which might appear as "sanctuary sites" providing a protective niche during antibiotic treatment.

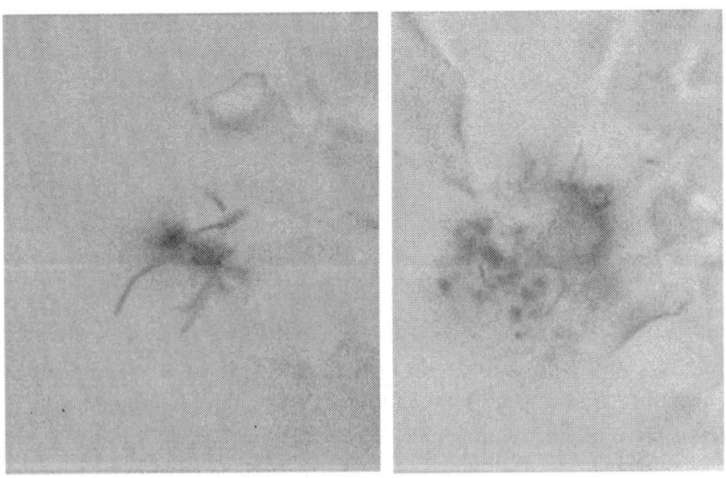

Figure 10. Borrelial colonies: "medusa colony" in a case of ACA (left) and "granular colony with a reddish veil" in a case of lichen sclerosus (right) shown by FFM (1000x).

As a possible underlying mechanism of immune evasion the inability of polymorphonucleates and monocytes to recognize unopsonized spirochetes has been postulated, suggesting that early persistence of spirochetes may be related to an inefficient clearance by phagocytic cells.

Another possible explanation for the resistance to antibiotic therapy in some patients with BL or ACA and the chronic relapsing courses of some borrelial infection could be the ability of *Borrelia* to form biofilm structures, however a definitive proof of biofilm formation by *Borrelia* is still missing. The biofilm hypothesis was recently proposed based on the finding of large colonies of *Borrelia* shown by immunohistochemistry and FFM. So, *Borrelia* can grow in a "medusa colony" or in a "granular colony with a reddish veil" (Figure 10). Biofilm formation makes the therapy difficult because in biofilms bacteria show much greater resistance to antibiotics than their free living counterparts.

On the other hand, well-performed prospective studies have found neither evidence of chronic infection nor a benefit worthy of long-term antibiotic therapy for these patients. Consequently, extended antibiotic therapy poses hazards, e.g. complications related to catheters, biliary disease, *Clostridium difficile* infection, and promotion of antibiotic resistance, therefore is not considered as acceptable [50-55].

In any case, considering that a 100% successfully treatment is generally not achievable (wrong adherence, compliance, immunosuppression), a low percentage of therapeutic failure is always to be expected, further, as in syphilis, reinfection might occur in highly endemic areas. On the other hand, a systemic infectious disease might trigger fatigue, depressive disorders or rheumatic diseases, or these frequent conditions could develop independently to the prior borrelial infection. Therefore, the decision how to treat these patients should be made by treating physician, based on the clinical findings and who should routinely review his own working hypothesis and treatment decision critically based on the patient's wellbeing.

References

[1] Steere, A. C. (2001). Lyme disease. *N Engl J Med.*, *345*(2), 115–9.

[2] Stanek, G., Wormser, G. P, Gray, J. & Strle, F. (2012). Lyme borreliosis. *Lancet.*, *379*(9814), 461-73.

[3] Deluca, J., Eisendle, K. & Zelger, B. (2013). Review On Cutaneous And Systemic Lyme Disease, *Expert Review of Dermatology*, in press.

[4] Müllegger, R. *Spirochätosen: Lyme-Borreliose, Leptospirose und Rückfallfieber. In: Braun-Falco's. Dermatologie, Venereologie und Allergologie*. SpringerVerlag. Chap. *14*, 199-211.

[5] Southwick, F. (2007). Zoonotic Infections. In: *Infectious disease: a clinical short course*. MacGraw Hill. New York. *13*, 322-328.

[6] Strle, F. (1999). Principles of the diagnosis and antibiotic treatment of Lyme borreliosis. *Wien Klin Wochenschr*, *111*(22-23), 911-5.

[7] Stanek, G. & Reiter, M. (2011). The expanding Lyme Borrelia complex-clinical significance of genomic species? *Clin Microbiol Infect*, *17*(4), 487-93.

[8] Dehnert, M., Fingerle, V., Klier, C., Talaska, T., Schlaud, M., Krause, G., Wilking, H. & Poggensee, G. (2012). Seropositivity of Lyme borreliosis and associated risk factors: a population-based study in Children and Adolescents in Germany (KiGGS). *PLoS One.*, 7(8), e41321

[9] Eisendle, K., Grabner, T. & Zelger, B. (2007). Focus floating microscopy: "gold standard" for cutaneous borreliosis? *Am J Clin Pathol*, *127*(2), 213-22.

[10] Fraser, C. M., Casjens, S. & Huang, W. M. (1997). *et al.* Genomic sequence of a Lyme disease spirochaete, Borrelia burgdorferi. *Nature*, *390*(6660), 580–86.

[11] Rizzoli, A., Hauffe, H., Carpi, G., Vourc, H. G., Neteler, M. & Rosa, R. (2011). Lyme borreliosis in Europe. *Euro Surveill*, *16*(27).

[12] Tsao, J. I. (2009). Reviewing molecular adaptations of Lyme borreliosis spirochetes in the context of reproductive fitness in natural transmission cycles. *Vet Res.*, 40(2), 36.

[13] Schwan, T. G., Piesman, J. & Golde, W.T. (1995). *et al.* Induction of an outer surface protein on Borrelia burgdorferi during tick feeding. *Proc Natl Acad Sci U S A.*, 92(7), 2909-13.

[14] de Silva, A. M. & Fikrig, E. (1997). Arthropod- and host-specific gene expression by Borrelia burgdorferi. *J Clin Invest.*, *99*, 377-9.

[15] Eisendle, K. & Zelger, B. (2009). The expanding spectrum of cutaneous borreliosis. *G Ital Dermatol Venereol.*, *144*(2), 157-71.

[16] Hofmann, H. (2005). Lyme-Borreliose. *Hautarzt.*, 56(8), 783–796.

[17] Müllegger, R. R. (2004). Dermatological manifestations of Lyme borreliosis. *Eur J Dermatol.*, 14(5), 296-309.

[18] Bhate, C. & Schwartz, R. A. (2011). Lyme disease: Part I. Advances and perspectives. *J Am Acad Dermatol.*, *64*(4), 619-36.

[19] Kirkland, K. B., Klimbo, T. B. & Meriwether, R. A., (1997). *et al.* Erythema migrans-like rash illness at a camp in North Carolina: a new tick-borne disease? *Arch Intern Med, 157*(22), 2635.

[20] Feder, H. M., Jr, Johnson, B. J. & O'connell, S. (2007). *et al.* Ad Hoc International Lyme Disease Group. A critical appraisal chronic Lyme disease. *N Engl J Med., 357*, 1422–30.

[21] Varela, A. S., Luttrell, M. P., Howerth, E.W., (2004). *et al.* First culture isolation of Borrelia lonestari, putative agent of southern tick-associated rash illness. *J Clin Microbiol., 42*(3), 1163–9.

[22] Oliveira, A., Fonseca, A. H., Costa, C. M., Mantovani, E., Yoshinari, N. H. (2010). Growth, cysts and kinetics of Borrelia garinii (Spirochaetales: Spirochaetacea) in different culture media. *Mem Inst Oswaldo Cruz, 105*(5), 717-9.

[23] Yoshinari, N. H., Mantovani, E., Bonoldi, V. L., Marangoni, R. G. & Gauditano, G. (2010). [Brazilian lyme-like disease or Baggio-Yoshinari syndrome: exotic and emerging Brazilian tick-borne zoonosis]. *Rev Assoc Med Bras., 56*(3), 363-9.

[24] Aberer, E., Neumann, R. & Stanek, G. (1985). Is localised scleroderma a Borrelia infection? *Lancet., 2*(8449), 278.

[25] Duray, P. H., Asbrink, E. & Weber, K. (1989). The cutaneous manifestations of human Lyme disease: a widening spectrum. *Adv Dermatol., 4*, 255-75.

[26] Aberer, E. & Stanek, G. (1987). Histological evidence for spirochetal origin of morphea and lichen sclerosus et atrophicans. *Am J Dermatopathol, 9*(5), 374-9.

[27] Eisendle, K., Grabner, T. & Zelger, B. (2007). Morphoea: a manifestation of infection with Borrelia species? *Br J Dermatol, 157*(6), 1189-98.

[28] Aberer, E., Schmidt, B. L., Breier, F. & Kinaciyan, Luger, A. (1999). Amplification of DNA of Borrelia burgdorferi in urine samples of patients with granuloma annulare and lichen sclerosus et atrophicus. *Arch Dermatol., 135*(2), 210-2.

[29] Eisendle, K., Baltaci, M., Kutzner, H. & Zelger, B. (2008). Detection of spirochaetal microorganisms by focus floating microscopy in necrobiosis lipoidica in patients from central Europe. *Histopathology, 52*(7), 877-84.

[30] Duray, P. H. (1989). Clinical pathologic correlations of Lyme disease. *Rev Infect Dis., 11*(6), 1487-93.

[31] Zelger, B., Eisendle, K. & Mensing, C. (2007). Detection of spirochetal micro-organisms by focus-floating microscopy in necrobiotic xanthogranuloma. *J Am Acad Dermatol.*, *57*(6), 1026-30.

[32] Ziemer, M., Eisendle, K., Müller, H. & Zelger, B. (2009). Lymphocytic infiltration of the skin (Jessner-Kanof) but not reticular erythematous mucinosis occasionally represents clinical manifestations of Borrelia-associated pseudolymphoma. *Br J Dermatol.*, *161*(3), 583-90.

[33] Ziemer, M., Eisendle, K. & Zelger, B. (2009). New concepts on erythema annulare centrifugum: a clinical reaction pattern that does not represent a specific clinicopathological entity. *Br J Dermatol*, *160*(1), 119-26.

[34] Eisendle, K., Grabner, T., Kutzner, H. & Zelger, B. (2008). Lichen sclerosus et atrophicus: a manifestation of infection with Borrelia species? *Arch Dermatol.*, *144*(5), 591-8.

[35] Weger, W. & Müllegger, R. R. (2011). Histopathology and immunohistochemistry of dermatoborrelioses. *Acta Dermatoven APA*, *10*,135-42.

[36] Grant-Kels, J. (2007). Nodular and Diffuse Dermatitis in: Color atlas of dermopathology. Informa Healthcare. New York. 8, 98.

[37] Wilske, B., Fingerle, V. & Schulte-Spechtel, U. (2007). Microbiological and serological diagnosis of Lyme borreliosis. *FEMS Immunol Med Microbiol*, *49*(1), 13-21.

[38] Garon, C. F., Dorward, D. W. & Corwin, M. D. (1989). Structural features of Borrelia burgdorferi--the Lyme disease spirochete: silver staining for nucleic acids. *Scanning Microsc Suppl.*, *3*,109-15.

[39] Aberer, E. (2007). Lyme borreliosis--an update. *J Dtsch Dermatol Ges.*, *5*(5), 406-14.

[40] Steere, A. C., McHugh, G., Damle, N. & Sikand, V. K. (2008). Prospective study of serologic tests for lyme disease. *Clin Infect Dis*, *47*(2), 188-95.

[41] Centers for Disease Control and Prevention (CDC). Recommendations for test performance and interpretation from the Second National Conference on Serologic Diagnosis of Lyme Disease. *MMWR Morb Mortal Wkly Rep*, *44* (31), 590-1 (1995).

[42] Brouqui, P., Bacellar, F., Baranton, G., (2004). *et al.* Guidelines for the diagnosis of tick-borne bacterial diseases in Europe. *Clin Microbiol Infect*, *10*(12), 1108-32.

[43] Dressler, F., Whalen, J. A., Reinhardt, B. N., Steere, A. C. (1993). Western blotting in the serodiagnosis of Lyme disease. *J Infect Dis, 167*(2), 392-400.

[44] Branda, J. A., Aguero-Rosenfeld, M. E. & Ferraro, M. J. (2010). *et al.* 2-tiered antibody testing for early and late Lyme disease using only an immunoglobulin G blot with the addition of a VlsE band as the second-tier test. *Clin Infect Dis., 50*(1), 20-6.

[45] Bhate, C. & Schwartz, R. A. (2011). Lyme disease: Part II. Management and prevention. *J Am Acad Dermatol.* 64(4), 639-53.

[46] Wormser, G. P., Dattwyler, R. J. & Shapiro, E. D. (2006). *et al.* The Clinical Assessment, Treatment, and Prevention of Lyme Disease, Human Granulocytic Anaplasmosis, and Babesiosis: Clinical Practice Guidelines by the Infectious Diseases Society of America. *Clin Infect Dis., 43*(9), 1089-134.

[47] Schutzer, S. E., Janniger, C. K. & Schwartz, R. A. (1991). Lyme disease during pregnancy. *Cutis, 47*(4), 267-8.

[48] MacDonald, A. B. (1986). Human fetal borreliosis, toxemia of pregnancy, and fetal death. *Zentralbl Bakteriol Mikrobiol Hyg A., 263*(1-2), 189–200.

[49] Lakos, A. & Solymosi, N. (2010). Maternal Lyme borreliosis and pregnancy outcome. *Int J Infect Dis., 14*(6), 494-8.

[50] Feder, H. M., Johnson, B. J. & O'Connell, S. (2007). *et al.* A critical appraisal of ''chronic Lyme disease''. *N Engl J Med., 357*(14), 1422–30.

[51] Mayer, L. & Merz, S. (2008). An appraisal of ''chronic Lyme disease''. *N Engl J Med., 358*(4), 428 (2008).

[52] Klempner, M. S. (2002). Controlled trials of antibiotic treatment in patients with post-treatment chronic Lyme disease. *Vector Borne Zoonotic Dis., 2*(4), 255-63.

[53] Shoberg, R. J. & Thomas, D. D. (1993). Specific adherence of Borrelia burgdorferi extracellular vesicles to human endothelial cells in culture. *Infect Immun., 61*(9), 3892-900.

[54] Sapi, E. & MacDonald, A. (2008). Biofilms of Borrelia burgdorferi in chronic cutaneous borreliosis. *Am J Clin Pathol., 129*, 988-9.

[55] Eisendle, K., Mueller, H. & Zelger, B. (2008). Biofilms of Borrelia burgdorferi in chronic cutaneous borreliosis. *Am J Clin Pathol, 129,* 989-90.

In: Dermatitis
Editor: Cornelia Sigrid Lissi Müller

ISBN: 978-1-62618-997-3

Chapter VI

Allergic Contact Dermatitis Associated with the Use of Orthodontic Appliances

Vanessa Paredes,[1,*] Rosa Cibrian[2] and Jose Luis Gandia[1]
[1] Orthodontics Department. University of Medicine and Dentistry. University of Valencia, Spain
[2]Physiology Department. University of Medicine and Dentistry. University of Valencia, Spain

Abstract

Allergic contact dermatitis (ACD) is a skin inflammation caused by an allergic reaction to contact with external substances small enough to be absorbed by the skin.

There are several studies describing allergic reactions, especially to nickel, caused by intraoral and extraoral orthodontic appliances. Nickel produces more allergic reactions than any other metal used in Orthodontics. It is estimated that between 2% to 27.5% of the general population are hypersensitive to nickel, females being affected more than males at a rate of 1/10. This allergy has increased with the more frequent use of jewellery and intraoral piercings containing nickel.

* Corresponding author. Dr. Vanessa Paredes, Clínica Odontológica. C/Gasco Oliag nº1 Valencia 46010, Valencia 46010 Spain. E-mail: vanessa.paredes@uv.es.

Allergic reactions due to intraoral appliances, as opposed to extraoral ones, are quite frequent. Extraoral reactions are also attributed to the metallic, elastic or textile components of extraoral appliances. ACD may involve clinical signs such as fissuring, desquamation, eczema, erythema, edema of the face or other skin areas and symptoms such as soreness and itching. The diagnosis of a nickel allergy is confirmed by patch testing.

This article provides a general review of all the different types of orthodontic braces that may cause ACD. Clinical cases of patients with this allergy are presented and guidelines provided for treating it. The importance of specific questioning particularly on sensitivity and previous allergic reactions when compiling medical records must be stressed, especially with female patients, as early diagnosis of this pathology is essential in order to achieve a total regression of the reaction. Orthodontists should be aware that ACD in predisposed patients can be caused by intraoral and extraoral orthodontic appliances. Alternative nickel-free treatments are recommended for the benefit of the patient.

Introduction

Orthodontists are sometimes required to treat patients with an allergy to nickel. This is a concern for the orthodontist because it is present in a vast array of materials frequently used in orthodontics. Nickel is the most common component both in intraoral and extraoral orthodontic appliances [1].

The response by the immune system to nickel is usually a Type IV cell mediated delayed hypersensitivity, also called an allergic contact dermatitis (ACD). It is mediated by T-cells and monocytes/macrophages rather than antibodies and consists of two phases. The first phase, or sensitization, occurs when nickel initially enters the body. There is usually no response present at this time, but the immune system is primed or sensitized for an allergic response. The major sensitization routes are nickel-containing jewellery and foods. Foods that are high in nickel include chocolate, soybeans, nuts and oatmeal. The response, or the elicitation phase, comes in the form of contact mucositis or dermatitis that occurs during re-exposure to nickel and develops over a period of days or rarely up to three weeks. If nickel is leached from orthodontic appliances, this Type IV hypersensitivity reaction can occur [1].

Etiology

The World health Organization defines adolescence as the period between 10 and 19 years. During those years, adolescents can present either irritative dermatitis or allergic contact dermatitis (ACD). ACD is due to the fact that, during these years, adolescents come into contact with various allergens; perfumes, piercings, tattoos and treatments with orthodontic appliances containing nickel, the main source of sensitization to nickel being produced by perforation of the pinna, in many countries at birth. For this reason allergy to nickel is most frequent in females, as girls wear earrings at earlier ages than boys and in both pinnae [2-3]. The fashion for piercings has led to an increase in allergy to this metal also among males. In fact, the risk of allergy to nickel increases with the number of piercings [4].

The second type of dermatitis, irritative one, is caused by woollen garments and footwear [2-3].

It must be borne in mind that adolescents that have suffered some kind of dermatitis during infancy, such as atopic dermatitis or psoriasis, are more susceptible to possible sensitizations, made easier by having had their cutaneous barrier altered or by having been in contact with topical treatments that are potential allergens [2-3].

When orthodontic appliance use preceded exposure to piercing, there is a reduced risk of nickel sensitivity. Furthermore, there is a reduced risk with the use of full fixed appliances with an assumed high release of nickel as compared with appliances including alloys with a lower nickel release [4].

The risk reduction is most prominent when the duration of orthodontic treatment (before piercing) is 1–2.5 years. These results should thus reduce parental and patient concerns about sensitization from orthodontic appliances. The results support the concept of induction of immunological tolerance via oral administration of nickel [4].

Prevalence and Pathogeny

To find out the prevalence of allergic contact dermatitis among adolescents is difficult as there are very few studies in which epicutaneous tests have been carried out and which evaluate the relevance of the positivity of these tests, although it is estimated at around 15%. If we take only orthodontic patients into account on considering the frequency of allergic reactions, it is claimed that about 1 per cent of the orthodontic population exhibits some kind of adverse reaction [5-6].

Most studies agree that there is a female predominance of contact dermatitis in adolescents, although the results are not statistically significant.

Nearly half of the respondents reported adverse patient reactions associated with orthodontic treatment during the last 5 years. The number of recalled adverse reactions was more than double in Finland compared with Norway, and headgear was most often attributed to the reaction, especially in Finland. More than half of the reactions had implications for the treatment. Although most respondents in both countries used nickel-containing fixed appliances regularly for patients who self-reported a nickel allergy, orthodontists in Norway tended to select nickel-free appliances more often for these patients [7].

Clinic

ACD can include the following extraoral and intraoral oral clinical signs and symptoms. Extraoral such as acute facial eczema with erythema, edema and vesiculacion and intraoral clinical signs and symptoms such as a burning sensation, gingival hyperplasia, labial desquamation, angular chelitis, erythema multiforme, periodontitis, stomatitis with mild to severe erythema, papular peri-oral rash, loss of taste or metallic taste, numbness, soreness at side of the tongue. It should be noted that symptoms could occur without signs. Extraoral manifestations of nickel allergy may have an intraoral origin [1].

Diagnosis

The diagnosis of a response to nickel in the oral mucosa is more difficult than on the skin. A known allergy to nickel should be determined when the patient completes the medical questionnaire or during a verbal medical history review [1].

Diagnosis is undertaken by means of epicutaneous tests, which pose no danger to the patients. The criteria for carrying out contact tests are when there is a clinical suspicion of contact allergy or dermatitis that does not evolve adequately. We must not carry out tests when the patient presents acute eczema due to the possibility of reactivating the eczema or producing false positives. We should also not use substances in the tests if we do not know their irritant or allergic capability, as we could cause active sensitizations or serious local reactions. Once the allergen that has caused the ACD has been identified, contact with it must be prevented. Patients must be warned what they are allergic to and how to avoid such substances. Extraoral irritation and hypersensitivity, with dermatitis on the face and neck, are the adverse patient reactions most commonly reported by orthodontists, but intraoral reactions are also frequent. Most of them are of moderate severity and treatment can be continued [6].

There are several studies describing allergic reactions, in particular to nickel [1, 7-8], due to intraoral orthodontic appliances. Nickel is a common component in many orthodontic materials. An allergic reaction to nickel is commonly found in the general population. This allergy has increased with the more frequent use of jewellery and intraoral piercings containing nickel [1]. Nickel is a common environmental allergen with approximately 10% of the female and 1% of the male population being sensitized [1, 9-10].

Allergic reactions due to extraoral appliances are not so frequent and there are relatively few studies on them. Extraoral reactions are attributed to metallic, elastic or textile parts of the extraoral appliances [11]. The irritant component of such reactions may be explained by friction between skin and the orthodontic appliance facilitated by sweat or saliva [12-15].

Treatment

If intra-oral and extraoral signs and symptoms are present and a diagnosis of nickel hypersensitivity is established, the nickel titanium orthodontic appliance should be removed and replaced with stainless steel archwire, which is low in nickel content.

All the patients should be seen by a dermatologist and cortisone pomade should be prescribed as a local treatment [16-17].

Description of Cases

We are now going to present 6 patients who had ACD due to the use of extraoral dental appliances. The patients mean age was between 9/1 and 11/7 years of age. All of them were attended a private orthodontic clinic in

Valencia, Spain, in order to receive orthodontic treatment. Their medical and dental records were non-contributory.

All of them presented mandibular prognathism. Due to this skeletal problem, rapid maxillary expansion was performed with a Hyrax appliance, while a Petit orthopaedic face mask was fitted. The patients were asked to wear the facemask for 12 to 14 hours a day in the evening and at night. The Petit facemask has two supports; one at the forehead and the other at the chin.

The lesions of allergic contact dermatitis (ACD) appeared at the points of contact with the facemask, i.e. on the chin, within a week of wearing the orthodontic appliance more or less. The lesions that we describe were of a wide-ranging nature.

Figures 1A and 1B show an irregular lesion, not well defined and reddish in color. In these two cases, the lesions did not cause any irritation to the patients, such as burning sensation.

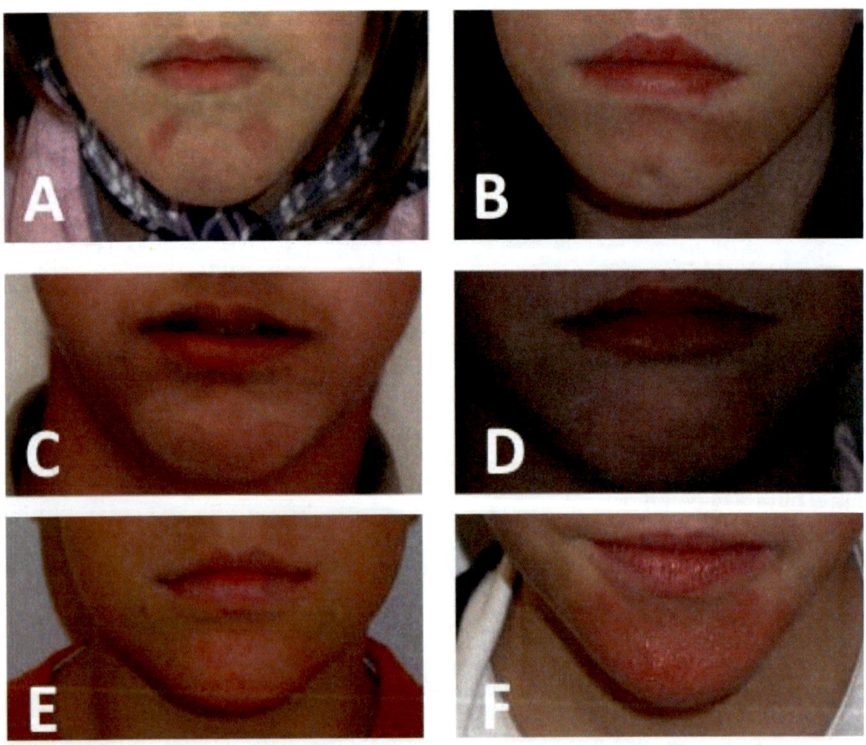

Figure 1.

In contrast, Figures 1C and 1D show facial eczema with erythema, and edema. It is a regular lesion, very well defined and whitish in color, much lighter than the skin color, and accompanied by desquamation. Just as in the two previous cases, no irritation to the patients, such as a burning sensation, was caused.

Lastly, Figures 1E and 1F show a regular lesion, very well defined, with a certain dark red swelling. In contrast to the four previous cases, these lesions caused irritation to the patients, such as a burning sensation.

All the patients were seen by a dermatologist, who prescribed cortisone pomade as a local treatment (Paredes V at al., 2010; Paredes at al., 2011). The use of the facemask was discontinued at this time. Treatment was effective and the lesions disappeared within 2 weeks.

At the end of this two-week period, it was decided that the patients should wear the facemask on alternate days with regular use of moisturising cream.

Conclusion

Allergic reactions are quite frequent, as was seen in a study carried out by orthodontists in Finland and Norway. Forty-six percent of those orthodontists had reported at least 1 adverse patient reaction over the previous 5 years [7].

Although most of the studies consulted in the literature describe allergic reactions to the nickel of intraoral appliances, a few studies also describe allergic contact dermatitis to manganese, evidenced by eczematous lesions in the dorsum of fingers and hands, and itching lesions in lips and oral cavity, due to the management of prosthetic material and orthodontics respectively [18] and others ACD due to extraoral appliances.

Notwithstanding the worldwide use of facemasks and the possible implication of extraoral appliances in the development of allergic contact dermatitis (ACD), no clinical reports were found in the literature. All the studies described allergic reactions to headgear, but not facemasks.

The irritant component of such reactions may be explained by friction between skin and parts of the orthodontic appliances [6]. One of the favourable factors in the development of ACD is humidity plus high temperatures, which provoke sweating in the support area of the facemask with the chin. Furthermore, the patient who is prone to atopic dermatitis was another ACD predisposing factor.

Though an allergic response to nickel in the oral mucosa from nickel containing orthodontic appliances is more infrequent than from nickel contact on the epidermis, it can occur, particularly in females. If nickel-related intraoral clinical signs and symptoms appear, the orthodontist should be prepared to undertake or continue treatment without the use of Ni-Ti wires and even without stainless steel. These two cases illustrate that clinical signs of nickel hypersensitivity may be subtle or absent. The frequency of orthodontic treatment and the common use of nickel containing orthodontic materials raises the interesting question of whether orthodontic treatment may act to increase or decrease the burden of nickel hypersensitivity in the population. There is evidence that oral exposure to nickel may induce immunologic tolerance to nickel and thereby reduce the incidence of nickel hypersensitivity causing distress to patients. There are many choices of materials available to the orthodontist as alternatives [1].

In conclusion, we can say that appliances containing nickel may not be tolerated well by nickel-hypersensitive patients. Dermatologists need to be aware of the allergenic materials used in orthodontics in order to correctly manage skin disease in this high-risk group.

These cases demonstrate the importance of specific questioning on, in particular, sensitivity and previous allergic reactions when compiling medical records, especially with female patients. This assessment is also supported by others authors in the literature.

Finally, it is essential that an early diagnosis of this pathology is made in order to obtain total regression of the allergic reaction. Orthodontists should be aware that ACD in predisposed patients could be caused by facemasks.

References

[1] Noble, J; Ahing, SI; Karaiskos, NE; Wiltshire, WA. Nickel allergy and orthodontics, a review and report of two cases. *Br Dent J.*, 2008, Mar 22, 204(6), 297-300.

[2] Gober, MD. DTJ; Gaspari, AA. Contact dermatitis. Jr AN, editor. Philadelphia, Pa: Mosby Elsevier, 2008, chap 632008.

[3] Habif, TP. Contact dermatitis and patch testing. . 5th ed. TP H, editor. Philadelphia, Pa: Mosby Elsevier, 2009.

[4] Fors, R; Persson, M; Bergstrom, E; Stenlund, H; Stymne, B; Stenberg, B. Lifestyle and nickel allergy in a Swedish adolescent population: effects of piercing, tattooing and orthodontic appliances. *Acta Derm Venereol.*, 2012, Oct, 92(6), 664-8.

[5] Jacobsen, N; Aasenden, R; Hensten-Pettersen, A. Occupational health complaints and adverse patient reactions as perceived by personnel in public dentistry. *Community Dent Oral Epidemiol.*, 1991, Jun, 19(3), 155-9.

[6] Jacobsen, N; Hensten-Pettersen, A. Occupational health problems and adverse patient reactions in orthodontics. *Eur J Orthod.*, 1989, Aug, 11(3), 254-64.

[7] Kerosuo, HM; Dahl, JE. Adverse patient reactions during orthodontic treatment with fixed appliances. *Am J Orthod Dentofacial Orthop.*, 2007, Dec, 132(6), 789-95.

[8] Kolokitha, OE; Chatzistavrou, E. A severe reaction to ni-containing orthodontic appliances. *Angle Orthod.*, 2009, Jan, 79(1), 186-92.

[9] Burden, DJ; Eedy, DJ. Orthodontic headgear related to allergic contact dermatitis: a case report. *Br Dent J.*, 1991, Jun, 22, 170(12), 447-8.

[10] Schuster, G; Reichle, R; Bauer, RR; Schopf, PM. Allergies induced by orthodontic alloys: incidence and impact on treatment. Results of a survey in private orthodontic offices in the Federal State of Hesse, Germany. *J Orofac Orthop.*, 2004, Jan, 65(1), 48-59.

[11] Jacobsen, N; Hensten-Pettersen, A. Changes in occupational health problems and adverse patient reactions in orthodontics from 1987 to 2000. *Eur J Orthod.*, 2003, Dec, 25(6), 591-8.

[12] Brooks, MH; Curzon, PG. 'Orthodontic headgear related to allergic contact dermatitis'. *Br Dent J.*, 1991, Sep 7, 171(5), 124.

[13] Dickson, G. Contact dermatitis and cervical headgear. *Br Dent J.*, 1983, Aug 20, 155(4), 112.

[14] Greig, DG. Contact dermatitis reaction to a metal buckle on a cervical headgear. *Br Dent J.*, 1983, Jul 23, 155(2), 61-2.

[15] Lowey, MN. Allergic contact dermatitis associated with the use of an Interlandi headgear in a patient with a history of atopy. *Br Dent J.*, 1993, Jul 24, 175(2), 67-72.

[16] Paredes, V; Paredes, C. Allergic contact dermatitis associated with the use of facemask on a patient with a history of atopy. *J Dent Child* (Chic)., 2010, Sep-Dec, 77(3), 177-9.

[17] Paredes, V; Zamora, N; Paredes, C. [Contact dermatitis associated with the use of extraoral orthodontic appliances: a presentation of 3 cases.]. *An Pediatr (Barc).* 2011, Dec 21.

[18] Velasquez, D; Zamberk, P; Suarez, R; Lazaro, P. Allergic contact dermatitis to manganese in a prosthodontist with orthodontics. *Allergol Immunopathol (Madr).* 2010, Jan-Feb;38(1), 47-8.

In: Dermatitis
Editor: Cornelia Sigrid Lissi Müller
ISBN: 978-1-62618-997-3

Chapter VII

T-Lymphocyte Clonality in Inflammatory Skin Diseases

Cornelia S. L. Müller*

The Saarland University Hospital, Department of Dermatology, Homburg/Saar, Germany

Abstract

One of the main challenges for dermatopathologists is to distinguish between benign and malignant inflammatory skin diseases on the basis of morphology; in several clinical, as well as histologic settings, this is difficult-to-impossible. Additionally, missing clinical information and small biopsies hamper the likelihood that a dermatopathologist will establish the correct diagnosis within a short interval of time. More than one biopsy is often needed and objective methods for distinguishing benign from malignant lesions are clearly needed. This chapter reviews the existing knowledge on T cell clonality in inflammatory skin diseases and demystifies the notion of having an ever-working tool for detection of malignant cutaneous lymphomatoid diseases in early stages of the disease.

* Corresponding author: Phone: 0049-6841-16-23795, Fax: 0049-6841-16 13816, Email: cornelia.mueller@uks.eu.

Introduction

Detection of clonal T cells by PCR for TCR-γ rearrangements and high-resolution electrophoresis has been routinely used for the diagnosis of cutaneous T cell lymphomas [1]. The primary indication for gene rearrangement studies is the differentiation of cutaneous T – cell lymphoma from reactive lymphoid T-cell infiltrates (pseudolymphomas; [2]). The clonal growth of T cells is the basis for the cellular immune system and occurs in all T cell-dependent immune reactions [1]. The following inflammatory skin diseases have been shown to harbor clonal T cells to a variable degree [2-4]:

- lichen planus
- pityriasis lichenoides chronica
- pityriasis lichenoides et varioliformis acuta (PLEVA; Mucha Haberman disease)
- persistent pigmented purpuric dermatitis
- cutaneous lymphoid hyperplasia/ pseudolymphoma

Based on a review of the current literature, additional inflammatory diseases are known to involve monoclonal T-cells, such as benign lichenoid keratosis and lichen sclerosus et atrophicus. In contrast, clonal T cells are rarely detected in classic inflammatory skin diseases (psoriasis vulgaris and allergic or toxic contact dermatitis; [1]).

Benign Lichenoid Keratosis

Benign lichenoid keratoses (BLK) are solitary skin lesions of unknown etiology, and for which the genetic basis is also unknown. Recently, Groesser *et al.* [5] showed that FGFR3, PIK3CA, and RAS mutations are present in approximately 50% of BLKs, a finding that supports the theory that at least a portion of BLKs represent regressive variants resulting from former benign epidermal tumors (seborrhoeic keratosis and solar lentigo). The morphology of BLK includes a band-like lymphohistiocytic infiltrate at the dermal-epidermal junction with numerous dyskeratotic keratinocytes. Clinically, BLK lesions present as round skin lesions, dusky violoaecous-to-pink in color, with a predominant distribution involving the trunk, upper extremities, and face [5]. The reported composition of the inflammatory infiltrate in BLKs differs between investigators; being however, CD3+ T cells with few B cells predominate [6], While other groups have shown a predominant CD4+ and CD8 +phenotype [7]. Indeed, the reported differences in the composition and immunophenotype of the inflammatory infiltrate in BLKs are thought to be dependent on the duration of the lesion. Smith et al. [9] reported CD8-positive T-cells within the infiltrate. Additionally, TCR-γ chain rearrangement studies on biopsies with BLK have revealed a polyclonal population of T cells [8].

Lichen Sclerosus et Atrophicus

Lichen sclerosus et atrophicus (LSA) is a chronic dermatosis of unknown etiology and pathogenesis [1]. The histopathology of LSA is characterized by a lichenoid infiltrate consisting mainly of T cells, thus resembling the morphology of early mycosis fungoides. A stage-dependent shift of CD3+ T cells from a CD4+ to a CD8+ phenotype can be observed in LSA; the higher the level of CD8-positivity, the greater the degree of epidermotropism and basal degeneration, which is caused by the expression of cytotoxic granules within the cytotoxic T cells. Lukowsky *et al.* [1] investigated 39 cases of LSA and reported that the presence of clonally-expanded T cells could not be assigned to the CD4 or CD8+ phenotype or the degree of epidermotropism in 49% of the cases [1]; no correlation with patient age, gender, disease stage, or localization was demonstrated [1].

Lichenoid Purpura

Lichenoid purpura, also known as pigmented purpuric dermatoses, is a common skin disease which is characterized by slightly erythematous purpuric macules and patches, and typically has a "cayenne pepper" appearance (Figure 1). Lichenoid purpura has a predilection for the lower extremities [9]. The histopathologic features of lichenoid purpura include a band-like lymphoid infiltrate with extravasation of erythrocytes and hemosiderin deposition. Development of lichenoid purpura into mycosis fungoides has been previously reported [9-12]. Boyd et al. [10] examined 7 patients with lichenoid purpura, and 43% of whom exhibited a monoclonal T cell population. Boyd et al. [10] concluded that the presence of monoclonal T cells is not synonymous with malignancy, but patients with lichenoid purpura must be followed for the possible development of mycosis fungoides; it cannot be presumed that lichenoid purpura is a self-limiting, harmless skin disease.

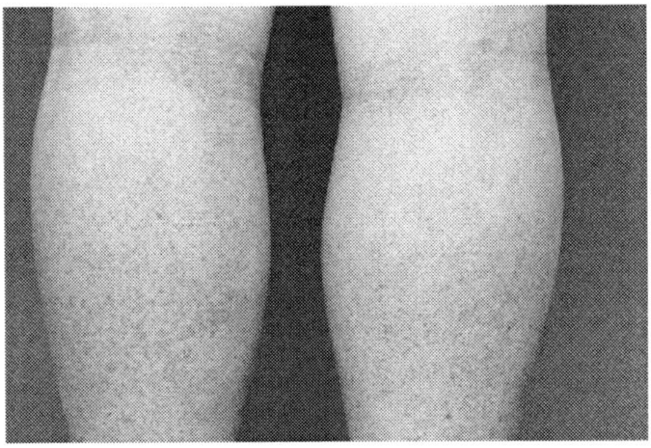

Figure 1. Typical cayenne pepper appearance of purpuric dermatoses.

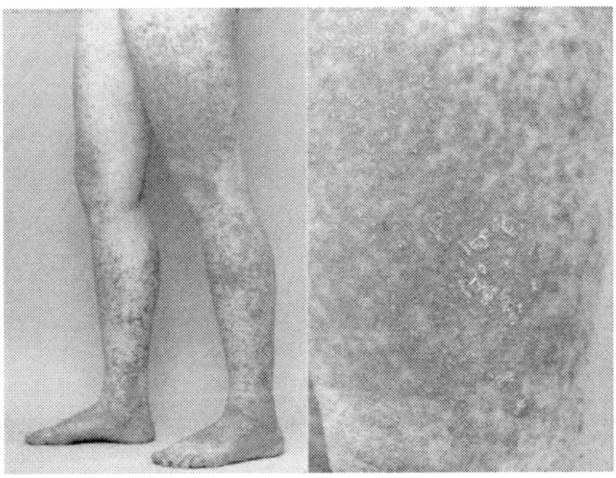

Figure 2. Exanthematic lichen planus (left: afar, right: closely).

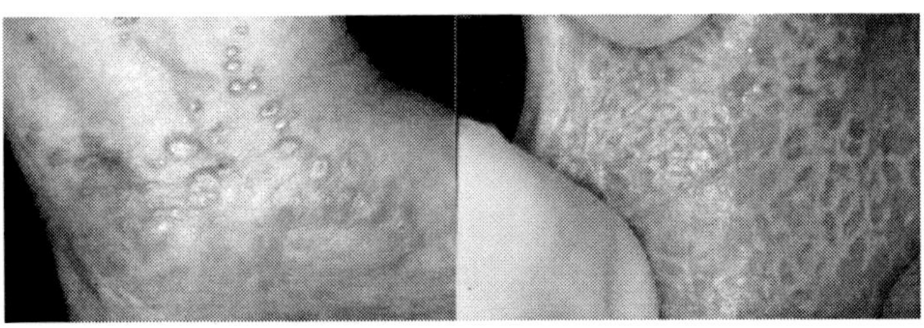

Figure 3. Characteristic lesions of lichen planus at the wrist (left) and oral lichen planus "Wickham sign" (right).

Lichen Planus

Lichen planus (LP) is a classic dermatologic condition of unknown origin affecting the skin, genital mucosa, scalp, and nails. LP is characterized by an intense pruritus of the skin and mucous membranes, is localized or systemic, and the main clinical feature are distinctive purple, flat-topped papules with a predilection for the trunk and flexor surfaces. Oral LP occurs in solation or in association with the outer skin (Figures 2 and 3). Oral LP follows a refractory course; affected patients experience immense pain and haphalgesia [3, 13-14]. Histopathologically, LP and oral LP are characterized by a band-like lymphocytic inflammatory infiltrate with exocytosis of lymphocytes and vacuolar degeneration of basal keratinocytes (cytotoxic interface dermatitis) and apoptosis [13]. Lesions involving the buccal mucosa are also known as the "Wickham sign" (white striae of the buccal mucosa; Figure 3). LP co-exists with hepatitis c and diabetes mellitus, but the clinical significance is a matter of debate. Schiller et al. [2] reported that 25% of all patients with LP had a monoclonal T-cell population within the inflammatory skin lesions; none of these patients developed malignant cutaneous lymphoma. Skewed T cell receptor (TCR) repertoires are found in tissue samples from patients with oral LP, and involvement of these T cells bearing these TCRs are involved in the pathogenesis of oral LP [13]. Sugerman et al. [16] detected several populations of clonal T cells within lesions of oral LP and discussed the role of "LP-specific T cells" within lesions of oral LP. The differential diagnosis for oral LP includes lichenoid reactions (lichenoid drug reactions or contact hypersensitivity; [15]).

Pityriasis Lichenoides

Pityriasis lichenoides (PL) is a rare inflammatory disease of unknown etiology with acute and chronic forms (Figure 4). Mucha-Habermann (pityriasis lichenoides et varioliformis acuta [PLEVA]) disease corresponds to the acute form of PL and is characterized by recurrent erythematous round papules, hemorrhage, blisters, and varioliform vesiculopustules with a variable distribution of the lesions; the scalp, hands, and feet are rarely involved. There may be a few episodes of PL and complete resolution within 6-8 weeks, but lesions may also recur over many months or even years. The chronic form of PL is called pityriasis lichenoides chronica (PLC). Currently, both the acute and chronic forms of PL are considered to be the extremes of a spectrum of cutaneous inflammatory diseases; concurrent or sequential occurrences in the same patient are known [15].

Kempf et al. [17] studied 13 cases of PLEVA with numerous CD30+ cells and demonstrated the following main immunophenotype: CD45RO+, CD2+, CD3+, CD8+, TIA-1+, Granzyme B-cells. The differential diagnosis of PLEVA includes lymphomatoid papulosis. Amongst the patients studied by Kempf et al. (17), only 55% had monoclonal T cells, while group reported that 57% of patients had monoclonal T-cell receptor gene arrangements [16]. Three main theories of pathogenesis of PLEVA have been advanced, as follows:

- Immune complex-mediated vasculitis theory. Supporting this theory, slight vascular depositions of IgM and C3 have been detected [17-19]. True lymphocytic vasculitis rarely occurs in patients with PLEVA. Leucocytoclastic vasculitis is also rare, but overrepresented in PLEVA [15, 18, 20]
- Inflammatory reaction triggered by an infectious agent. Immunologic or hypersensitivity reaction against an infectious agent leads to subsequent activation of TCR-restricted effector cytotoxic T-cells, although the causative infectious agent has not been determined [21]. Parvovirus B19 appears to be pathogenically-linked to PLEVA; however, it is not clear if parvovirus B19 is a true pathogen or an innocent bystander [15, 22].
- PLEVA as a lymphoproliferative disorder (designated as a T-cell dyscrasia). The occurrence of clonal T-cells supports the theory that PLEVA is a lymphoproliferative disorder. The monoclonality occurs in 10% of all patients with PLEVA [22].

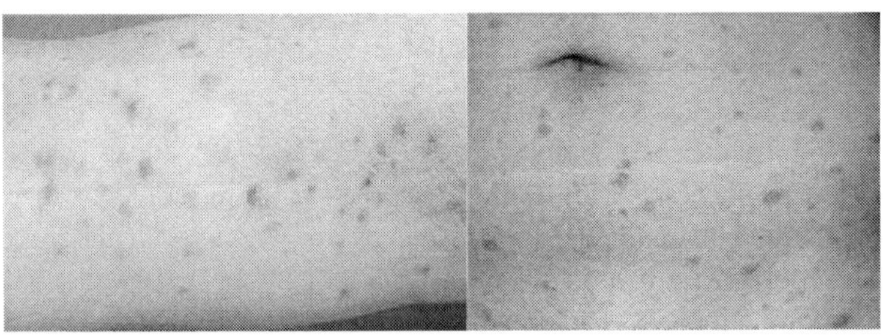

Figure 4. Pityriasis lichenoides chronica (left) and pityriasis lichenoides et varioliformis acuta (right).

Interestingly, and in contrast to the findings in patients with PLEVA, PL chronica has been shown to harbor a polyclonal T-cell rich inflammatory infiltrate [16]. Hence, it has been proposed that PLEVA is a benign clonal T-cell disorder, a clone that arises from a subset of T cells in lesions of PL chronica [16]. Another group has proposed that PL is a form of indolent cutaneous lymphoid dyscrasia and limited progression to classical mycosis fungoides may reflect internal mechanisms of controlling T cell clones via CD8 and CD4/25+ regulatory T cells [23]. Magro et al. [27] concluded that PLRVA and PL chronica are not two extremes of a single benign reactive dermatoses, but a spectrum of pre-malignant T cell dyscrasias.

Lupus Erythematosus Panniculitis

Lupus erythematosus panniculitis (LEP) or lupus profundus is a type of lupus erythematosus characterized by deep dermal or subcutaneous nodules, most often involving the head, face, or upper arms. LEP is generally chronic and occurs most often in middle-aged women. The differential diagnosis includes subcutaneous panniculitis-like T-cell lymphoma (SPTCL; 28. The diagnosis of LPE is difficult in cases in which involvement of the subcutaneous fat is the only manifestation of the disease [24]. In a case series, Park et al. [29] reported that 10% of patients with LPE exhibited monoclonality. In contrast, Magro et al. [30] reported monoclonality in 64.3% of patients with LPE and stated that this is associated with clinical and histopathologic atypical features, and Massone et al. [28] reported a polyclonal TCR gamma rearrangement. The most challenging differential diagnosis in patients with LPE is lymphoma within the panniculitis. In summary, clonality cannot be used as a discriminating feature of LEP and subcutaneous panniculitis-like T-cell lymphoma alone; clinical presentation, histopathologic features, and immunohistochemistry and molecular studies must be taken together to establish a correct diagnosis.

Kimura's Disease

Kimura's disease is a chronic, inflammatory disease of unknown etiology that is rare in Western countries, but endemic in Asia [25]. The clinical features of Kimura's disease involve painful and pruritic solitary or multiple subcutaneous, slowly enlarging nodules. Kimura's disease is often accompanied by regional lymphadenopathy, elevated serum eosinophil counts, and markedly elevated serum immunoglobulin E levels [25]. There have been no reports of malignant transformation of Kimura`s disease to malignant lymphoproliferative disorders [26]. Histologically, the lesions are characterized by reactive lymphoid follicles with eosinophilic infiltration and an increased number of post-capillary venules [25]. Kimura's disease has been interpreted as a reactive condition because two case series have shown no evidence of T cell clonality [27-28].

In contrast, Chim et al. [32] reported a case of Kimura`s disease in a 62-year old male patient with clonal T cell receptor rearrangement within the initial lesions and recurrent lesions 3 years after the primary biopsy. Like idiopathic eosinophilia, which is due to overproduction of interleukin-5 by clonal T cells, the hypereosinophilia in Kimura`s disease can be triggered by clonal T cell populations [26].

Granulomatous Disorders

Granulomatous mycosis fungoides (GMF) is the best known malignant lymphoma of the skin that exhibits a predominant granulomatous atypical infiltrate. GMF was first described by Ackerman and Flaxman in 1970 [35], and is characterized by distinct clinical and microscopice features. A major pitfall in the daily routine work of dermatopathologists is overlooking the diagnosis of mycosis fungoides in the presence of secondary granulomatous infiltration.

A granulomatous infiltrate can be observed in cutaneous T-cell lymphoma, and less frequently in cutaneous B-cell lymphoma [29]. A comprehensive study by Dabiri et al. [36] enumerated the frequency of T-cell clonality in association with granulomatous dermatitides and found one case of necrobiotic xanthogranuloma harboring clonal T-cells, whereas granuloma annulare, granulomatous drug-reaction, sarcoidosis, leprosy, and non-Langerhans cell histiocytosis did not reveal T cell clonality.

It is important to be aware of the possibility of a "pseudolymphomatous" variant of granuloma annulare, which represents another important pitfall in the morphologic diagnosis of this disease that could lead to misinterpretation and overtreatment as a malignant lymphoproliferative disorder [30].

Pseudolymphoma

Pseudolymphomas are defined as cellular infiltrates composed mainly of T and/ or B-lymphocytes with a variable admixture of non-lymphoid cells (eosinophils or neutrophils; [38]). The main challenge in evaluating patients with pseudolymphomas is to distinguish pseudolymphomatous reactive infiltrates from original cutaneous malignant lymphomas [31]. Several infectious disorders are known to induce dense lymphoid infiltrates simulating cutaneous lymphomas based on histopathologic evaluation: viral warts; herpes simplex; herpes zoster; molluscum contagiosum; and mycozic infections with dermatophytes [31]. Of note, even the diagnosis of scabies is not always a simple process based on clinical examination without the detection of mites; indeed, the histologic findings can be difficult, particularly without a clinico-pathologic correlation. Stanisz et al. [40] presented a case of pseudolymphoamtous scabies that was detected in repeated skin biopsies after detection of the mites.

The following criteria are used to recognized a pseudolymphoma and avoid misdiagnosis and overtreatment [32]:

Clinical Presentation and Histopathological Features

Skin areas that are exposed to exogenous stimuli (e.g., insect bites) are more suggestive of pseudolymphomatous reactions. Hence, the clinical presentation is not very useful to distinguish benign from malignant lesions, as ulcerations are usually thought to be a sign of malignancy; however, insect bites are ulcerated or severe erythroderma occur not only in lymphomas as HIV-related CD8+ cutaneous T-cell lymphoma also manifests as erythroderma with lymphadenoathia. Co-existing clinical features, personal history, and follow-up features in conjunction with histopathologic findings provide a major opportunity to detect malignancy [32].

Immunophenotype

To date, an etiologic marker has not been identified that distinguishes between reactive or true malignant infiltrates. The aberrant expression or loss of expression of antigens of mature T lymphocytes (CD2, CD3, and CD5) correlates with T lymphocyte malignancies [32]).

Molecular Tools

The major focus of this chapter is characterization of current knowledge on clonal T lymphocytes in the context of inflammatory skin diseases. Currently, polymerase chain reactions are used to determine the clonality status of the skin. Clonality analysis must be critically used and always used in conjunction with all other patient data available.

Search for Causative Factors

The diagnosis of pseudolymphoma requires identification of causative etiologic factors. T-cell pseudolymphoma can be drug-induced (localized and diffuse forms are known), UV-induced (chronic actinic dermatitis), HIV-related, insect bite reactions or idiopathic.

B-cell pseudolymphomas are mainly Borrelia- or varizella zoster virus-related, vaccination induced or secondary to tattoos, drug induced, or idiopathic.

Summarizing, in all cases of pseudolymphomas, especially in those cases without a known etiologic factor, long-term follow-up of patients is urgently needed with repeated skin biopsies to detect transition to malignant lymphoid infiltrates.

Conclusion

Determination of clonality was originally thought to be a reliable method to distinguish whether or not a cutaneous lymphocytic infiltrate is benign or malignant. However, as presented in this chapter, monoclonality is not a good single criterion for malignancy and vice versa [33-34]. In fact, T cell receptor rearrangement studies have mainly served as adjuncts to assist in establishing correct diagnoses in several distinct clinical settings.

This chapter provides a comprehensive summary on several inflammatory diseases that exhibit T cell clonality to varying degrees. Most of these inflammatory diseases are benign, but aesthetically annoying and are far away from being a malignant lymphoid disorder. For dermatopathologists, clinicopathologic correlations in daily routine work are mandatory and of importance to the possibility of T cell clonality as occasional features of inflammatory skin diseases that are characterized by dense lymphocytic infiltrates. Thus, differentiation of early forms of cutaneous T cell lymphomas from benign inflammatory diseases with T cell clones remains a major challenge for every dermatologist and dermatopathologist.

References

[1] Lukowsky, A; Muche, JM; Sterry, W; Audring, H. Detection of expanded T cell clones in skin biopsy samples of patients with lichen sclerosus et atrophicus by T cell receptor-gamma polymerase chain reaction assays. *J Invest Dermatol.*, 2000, Aug, 115(2), 254-9.

[2] Dereure, O; Levi, E; Kadin, ME. T-Cell clonality in pityriasis lichenoides et varioliformis acuta: a heteroduplex analysis of 20 cases. *Arch Dermatol.*, 2000, Dec, 136(12), 1483-6.

[3] Schiller, PI; Flaig, MJ; Puchta, U; Kind, P; Sander, CA. Detection of clonal T cells in lichen planus. *Arch Dermatol Res.*, 2000, Nov, 292(11), 568-9.

[4] Shieh, S; Mikkola, DL; Wood, GS. Differentiation and clonality of lesional lymphocytes in pityriasis lichenoides chronica. *Arch Dermatol.*, 2001, Mar, 137(3), 305-8.

[5] Laur, WE; Posey, RE; Waller, JD. Lichen planus-like keratosis. A clinicohistopathologic correlation. *J Am Acad Dermatol.*, 1981, Mar, 4(3), 329-36.

[6] Akasu, R; From, L; Kahn, HJ. Lymphocyte and macrophage subsets in active and inactive lesions of lichen planus. *Am J Dermatopathol.*, 1993, Jun, 15(3), 217-23.

[7] Gadenne, AS; Strucke, R; Dunn, D; Wagner, M; Bleicher, P; Bigby, M. T-cell lines derived from lesional skin of lichen planus patients contain a distinctive population of T-cell receptor gamma delta-bearing cells. *J Invest Dermatol.*, 1994, Sep, 103(3), 347-51.

[8] Smith, DI; Vnencak-Jones, CL; Boyd, AS. T-lymphocyte clonality in benign lichenoid keratoses. *J Cutan Pathol.*, 2002, Nov, 29(10), 623-4.

[9] Boyd, AS; Vnencak-Jones, CL. T-cell clonality in lichenoid purpura: a clinical and molecular evaluation of seven patients. *Histopathology.*, 2003, Sep, 43(3), 302-3.

[10] Barnhill, RL; Braverman, IM. Progression of pigmented purpura-like eruptions to mycosis fungoides: report of three cases. *J Am Acad Dermatol.*, 1988, Jul, 19(1 Pt 1), 25-31.

[11] Cather, JC; Farmer, A; Jackow, C; Manning, JT; Shin, DM; Duvic, M. Unusual presentation of mycosis fungoides as pigmented purpura with malignant thymoma. *J Am Acad Dermatol.*, 1998, Nov, 39(5 Pt 2), 858-63.

[12] Toro, JR; Sander, CA; LeBoit, PE. Persistent pigmented purpuric dermatitis and mycosis fungoides: simulant, precursor, or both? A study by light microscopy and molecular methods. *Am J Dermatopathol.*, 1997, Apr, 19(2), 108-18.

[13] Gotoh, A; Hamada, Y; Shiobara, N; Kumagai, K; Seto, K; Horikawa, T; et al. Skew in T cell receptor usage with polyclonal expansion in lesions of oral lichen planus without hepatitis C virus infection. *Clin Exp Immunol.*, 2008, Nov, 154(2), 192-201.

[14] Ismail, SB; Kumar, SK; Zain, RB. Oral lichen planus and lichenoid reactions: etiopathogenesis, diagnosis, management and malignant transformation. *J Oral Sci.*, 2007, Jun, 49(2), 89-106.

[15] Kempf, W; Kazakov, DV; Palmedo, G; Fraitag, S; Schaerer, L; Kutzner, H. Pityriasis lichenoides et varioliformis acuta with numerous CD30(+) cells: a variant mimicking lymphomatoid papulosis and other cutaneous lymphomas. A clinicopathologic, immunohistochemical, and molecular biological study of 13 cases. *Am J Surg Pathol.*, 2012, Jul, 36(7), 1021-9.

[16] Weinberg, JM; Kristal, L; Chooback, L; Honig, PJ; Kramer, EM; Lessin, SR. The clonal nature of pityriasis lichenoides. *Arch Dermatol.*, 2002, Aug, 138(8), 1063-7.

[17] Clayton, R; Haffenden, G. An immunofluorescence study of pityriasis lichenoides. *Br J Dermatol.*, 1978, Nov, 99(5), 491-3.

[18] Muhlbauer, JE; Bhan, AK; Harrist, TJ; Moscicki, RA; Rand, R; Caughman, W; et al. Immunopathology of pityriasis lichenoides acuta. *J Am Acad Dermatol.*, 1984, May, 10(5 Pt 1), 783-95.

[19] Nieboer, C; Kalsbeek, GL. Immunofluorescence findings in pityriasis lichenoides. *Br J Dermatol.*, 1980, Jul, 103(1), 120-1.

[20] Clayton, R; Haffenden, G; Du Vivier, A; Burton, J; Mowbray, J. Pityriasis lichenoides--an immune complex disease. *Br J Dermatol.*, 1977, Dec, 97(6), 629-34.

[21] Bowers, S; Warshaw, EM. Pityriasis lichenoides and its subtypes. *J Am Acad Dermatol.*, 2006, Oct, 55(4), 557-72, quiz 73-6.

[22] Tomasini, D; Tomasini, CF; Cerri, A; Sangalli, G; Palmedo, G; Hantschke, M; et al. Pityriasis lichenoides: a cytotoxic T-cell-mediated

skin disorder. Evidence of human parvovirus B19 DNA in nine cases. *J Cutan Pathol.*, 2004, Sep, 31(8), 531-8.
[23] Magro, CM; Crowson, AN; Morrison, C; Li, J. Pityriasis lichenoides chronica: stratification by molecular and phenotypic profile. *Hum Pathol.*, 2007, Mar, 38(3), 479-90.
[24] Park, HS; Choi, JW; Kim, BK; Cho, KH. Lupus erythematosus panniculitis: clinicopathological, immunophenotypic, and molecular studies. *Am J Dermatopathol.*, 2010, Feb, 32(1), 24-30.
[25] Guimaraes, CS; Moulton-Levy, N; Sapadin, A; Vidal, C. Kimura's Disease. *Case Report Med.*, 2009, 424053.
[26] Chim, CS; Fung, A; Shek, TW; Liang, R; Ho, WK; Kwong, YL. Analysis of Clonality in Kimura's Disease. *Am J Surg Pathol.*, 2002, Aug, 26(8), 1083-6.
[27] Chim, CS; Shek, W; Liang, R; Kowng, YL. Kimura's disease: no evidence of clonality. *Br J Ophthalmol.*, 1999, Jul, 83(7), 880-1.
[28] Jang, KA; Ahn, SJ; Choi, JH; Sung, KJ; Moon, KC; Koh, JK; et al. Polymerase chain reaction (PCR) for human herpesvirus 8 and heteroduplex PCR for clonality assessment in angiolymphoid hyperplasia with eosinophilia and Kimura's disease. *J Cutan Pathol.*, 2001, Aug, 28(7), 363-7.
[29] Dabiri, S; Morales, A; Ma, L; Sundram, U; Kim, YH; Arber, DA; et al. The frequency of dual TCR-PCR clonality in granulomatous disorders. *J Cutan Pathol.*, 2011, Sep, 38(9), 704-9.
[30] Cota, C; Ferrara, G; Cerroni, L. Granuloma annulare with prominent lymphoid infiltrates ("pseudolymphomatous" granuloma annulare). *Am J Dermatopathol.*, 2012, May, 34(3), 259-62.
[31] Kash, N; Ginter-Hanselmayer, G; Cerroni, L. Cutaneous mycotic infections with pseudolymphomatous infiltrates. *Am J Dermatopathol.*, 2010, Jul, 32(5), 514-7.
[32] Bachelez, H. The uncertain status of cutaneous pseudolymphoma. *Actas Dermosifiliogr.*, 2009, Nov, 100 Suppl 1, 33-7.
[33] Flaig, MJ; Schuhmann, K; Sander, CA. Impact of molecular analysis in the diagnosis of cutaneous lymphoid infiltrates. *Semin Cutan Med Surg.*, 2000, Jun, 19(2), 87-90.
[34] Kohler, S; Zehnder, JL. Use of the polymerase chain reaction in the evaluation of cutaneous T-cell infiltrates. *Dermatol Clin.*, 1999, Jul, 17(3), 657-66, x.

In: Dermatitis
Editor: Cornelia Sigrid Lissi Müller
ISBN: 978-1-62618-997-3

Chapter VIII

Calcium Signalling in Inflammatory Skin Disease

Hedwig Stanisz *
The Saarland University Hospital, Department of Dermatology, Homburg/ Saar, Germany

Abstract

Calcium signaling is an universal mechanism of transduction and processing of information inside and between human cells. Ca2+ ions are second messengers responsible for many vital physiological functions such as proliferation, differentiation and cytokine secretion. A multitude of genes encode for proteins that form receptors, channels, transporters, pumps and chelators which control the cellular Ca2+ homeostasis. Genetic defects of some of these Ca2+ handling proteins cause, among others, impaired function of the immune system (severe combined immunodeficiency) or dyskeratosis of the skin (Morbus Darier). A lot is known about the role of Ca2+ in immune and skin cells. However, how Ca2+ signals affect inflammatory skin diseases is less clear. Therefore, the interplay between the cells of the immune system and the skin cells, in particular in cutaneous inflammation, will be summarized and discussed in the following chapter.

* Phone: 0049-6841-16-23836, Fax: 0049-6841-16 23845, Email: hedwig.stanisz@uks.eu.

Introduction

Given that cells of the human body form all together a functional unit intense communication between them has to take place to create reasonable interplay. For this, intercellular communication messenger systems are crucial. The plasma membrane in general forms a barrier between the intracellular and the extracellular space. Signals from the cell out and vice versa have to cross the plasma membrane. Certain molecules such as hormones have, due to their lipophilicity, the ability to cross the plasma membrane via diffusion and their message reaches the cell by intracellular receptors. Other molecules need receptors on the plasma membrane to be able to transmit their signal. The engagement of plasma membrane receptors results in the activation of signaling cascades leading to secretion of second messengers. Such ubiquitous second messengers in many human cells are the cyclic nucleotides c-AMP and the calcium ions. As a second messenger calcium is involved in a multitude of cellular processes ranging from cellular motility, over activation of enzymes, cell proliferation and migration, to cell death by apoptosis and even necrosis. The effects of calcium as a second messenger are tightly connected with its intracellular and even subcellular concentration. Generalized, cells have two major ways of manipulating their intracellular calcium concentration. One option is transport of calcium across the plasma membrane by specialized channels and pumps while the other is the release or uptake by the intracellular calcium stores and buffers. The most prominent plasma membrane calcium permeable ion channels are the voltage-gated calcium channels, receptor operated calcium channels (i.e. transient receptor potential (TRP) channels) and calcium release activated calcium (CRAC) channels encoded by Orai1, Orai2 and Orai3. The major intracellular calcium store is the endoplasmic reticulum (ER). However, other organelles such as mitochondria or melanosomes also play an important role in uptake and release of cytosolic calcium. Given that multitude of extracellular events that translate into an increase of cytosolic calcium exist, not only the amount of transported calcium matters for proper cellular response. The concert of repetitions, duration, amplitude, uptake and release of calcium is crucial to translate into a specific message that than results in a further functional outcome. For example, one could compare the dynamic changes in intracellular calcium signals with the Morse alphabet.

However, calcium is not only essential for proper function of many cellular signaling processes. A variety of enzymes, transcription factors and other proteins also need calcium as cofactor essential for their accurate functioning.

In this context, the endoplasmic reticulum not only plays a role in storage of calcium but also creates a calcium dependent milieu that allows proper protein transformation and trafficking via calcium binding chaperone proteins. As already mentioned, the endoplasmic reticulum serves as an important source of intracellular calcium. This organelle has the ability of rapidly releasing calcium into the cytosol after activation of inositol3-phosphate (IP3) or ryanodine receptors (RYR). For removing calcium from the cytosol the calcium-ATPase (PMCA) plays a major role. Furthermore, the sodium-calcium-exchanger as well as the sodium-calcium-potassium exchanger can also contribute in expulsing calcium from the intracellular space. In the ER the sarco-endoplasmatic-calcium-ATPases (SERCA) is the main mechanism to uptake calcium from the cytosol. The uptake of calcium from cytosol into mitochondria is still not that clear. Recent finding indicate a major role for mitochondrial Ca2+ uniporter protein and its activator MICU1 in this process. Given that mitochondria play an important role in modifying the activity of at least the Orai calcium channels, these findings can be of essential importance not only for the energy supply of the cell but also for all processes dependent on calcium entry across the plasma membrane [1-6].

Calcium Signaling in Keratinocytes

It is well known that intra- and extracellular calcium is crucial for proper keratinocyte function. The epidermis, where the keratinocytes are located, has a calcium gradient that is below the serum levels in the basal layers and rises to high calcium levels in the granular layer. This extracellular calcium gradient is essential for physiological proliferation and differentiation of these skin cells. In addition, a gradual rise in intracellular calcium is crucial for keratinocyte development. It has already been described that a so called calcium switch to intracellular calcium levels above 0.1 mM is a crucial for initiation of keratinocyte differentiation. The mechanisms that lead to this calcium switch are however not fully elucidated. There are strong indications that store operated calcium entry via CRAC channels play an important role in this physiological process. Activation of several plasma membrane based G-protein coupled receptors leads to an intracellular increase in of IP3 which leads to depletion of calcium from the ER stores. The decreased ER calcium concentration is sensed by the ER calcium sensors STIM1 and STIM2 with a change of their conformation state and subsequent movement towards the plasma membrane. Thus, STIM proteins interact with Orai channels leading to their opening and hence initiation of calcium entry across the plasma membrane. This calcium entry is abolished by reuptake of intracellular calcium into the endoplasmic reticulum by the SERCA pumps and by removing the calcium ions across the plasma membrane via the PMCAs. In addition of endothelin receptors certain cytokines such as Interleukin-31 and Interleukin-8 lead to an increase of the intracellular calcium concentration and are able to activate the CRAC channels. In keratinocytes this leads to release of β-endorphin and activation of signal transducer and activator of transcription 3 (STAT3). TRPC channels have been identified as alternative mechanism of calcium entry in keratinocytes and have directly been linked to cellular proliferation and differentiation. The release of interleukin-1α as well as interleukin-6, prostaglandins and ATP are also calcium dependent processes (Figure 1).

Given the importance of calcium signaling for keratinocyte function it is no surprise that genetic mutations that lead to an impaired or diminished function of calcium handling proteins such as SERCA2 cause pathological defects such as dyskeratinisation in diseases such as Morbus Darier and Morbus Hailey Hailey. It has been suggested that decreased calcium concentration in the ER leads to a missfolding or missprocessing of proteins involved in keratinocyte adhesion such as catherines. However, how impaired SERCA2 function impacts store operated calcium entry and the CRAC channel function has not been investigated so far [5, 7-18].

Calcium Signals in Melanocytes

Melanocytes present a minority in the epidermis. Nevertheless, they play crucial role in the communication network of the skin and are involved in the cutaneous response to stress. Changes in [Ca2+]i are important determinants for proper melanocyte function. High [Ca2+]i is required for active transport of L-phenylalanine into melanocytes by the calmodulin-dependent Ca2+-ATPase as well as for its turnover to L-tyrosine, an essential signaling event in melaninproduction. Furthermore, it has been shown that melanin binds Ca2+ and thereby regulates the redox state of melanocytes to prevent cell damage by oxidative stress. Moreover microphthalmia-associated transcription factor regulates the expression of multiple genes involved in melanogenesis and melanocyte survival such as tyrosinase, TRP1 and 2, Bcl2, and CDK2. Concomitant production of diacylglycerol together with a rise in intracellular calcium activate protein kinases that via phosphorylation of Raf-1 activate mitogen-activated protein kinase signaling pathways and CRE-binding protein-dependent phosphorylation of microphthalmia-associated transcription factor and its subsequent upregulation. Recently, endothelin-1 released from keratinocytes after UV radiation or during inflammation was shown to induce activation of CRAC channels in melanocytes. In addition, ET-1-induced phosphorylation of CRE-binding protein as well as the scaffold protein kinase suppressor of Ras (KSR2) activation of ERK cascade are calcium-dependent processes. There are also reports about the role of TRP channels such as TRPM1 for Ca2+ influx across the plasma membrane in human melanocytes suggesting an impact on melanin production in human melanocytes [4, 13, 19-20] (Figure 1).

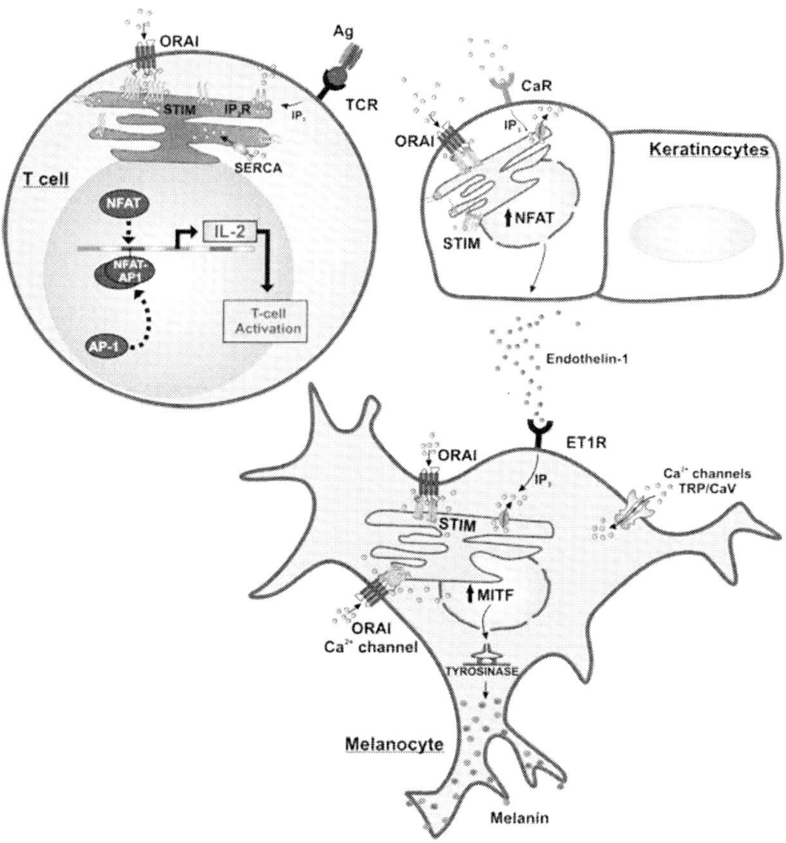

Figure 1. The role of STIM and ORAI proteins in calcium signaling of keratinocytes, melanocytes and T-cells.

Calcium Signaling in Mast Cells

Mast cells are known to play a major role in type I hypersensitivity reactions such as anaphylactic reactions, rhinoconjunctivitis and asthma. As immediate reaction on activation usually by engagement of the IgE-Receptor mast cells degranulate and liberate histamine and TNF-alpha as well as arachidonic acid-derived lipid mediators (prostaglandins and leukotriens). Prolonged effects of mast cell activation result in a secretion of cytokines that attract inflammatory cells such as granulocytes. Cross-linking of the IgE-Receptor FceR1 is the key event of mast cell degranulation and results in store operated calcium entry. Calcium entry into the mast cell is crucial for mast cell degranulation and liberation of histamine and other mediators. Gene expression and the arachidonic acid and leucotriene synthesis in mast cells are also calcium dependent. It is worth mentioning that not the overall change in intracellular calcium, but the so-called calcium microdomains seem to be crucial for proper mast cell function. Microdomains are due to localized calcium entry by for example CRAC channels which lead to a localized rise of intracellular calcium in a certain area of the cell. These microdomains and the associated shape and kinetics of the calcium signals translate the extracellular signal to an according reaction of the cell [2, 21-23].

Calcium Signaling in T-Cells

T-cells play a crucial role for the adaptive immune response. However, their missfunction leads to development of inflammatory skin diseases such as irritant or allergic contact dermatitis, atopic dermatitis as well as psoriasis.

T-cell activation requires the involvement of the T-cell-receptor. Upon formation of the immunological synapse and the antigen presentation, IP3 is secreted leading to activation of Orai channels via the above described signaling cascade. Dependent on the T-cell subtype (TH1, TH2 or TH17) the calcium signals differ and lead to a specific production of cytokines. The increase in intracellular calcium activates the calcineurin and the calcium-calmodulin kinase pathways and leads to translocation of nuclear factor of activated T-cells (NFAT) into the nucleus. These transcription factors can than bind to DNA binding sites in the promoter of target genes.

Most often NFAT is associated with other transcription factors for initiating the transcription of defined genes in T-cell subsets. NFAT regulates numerous genes responsible for T-cell-development and T-cell-effector function [3-4, 6, 24] (Figure 1).

Atopic Dermatitis and Calcium

Impaired skin barrier function is supposed to play a major role in the pathophysiology of atopic dermatitis. It was shown that the impaired skin barrier goes along with a loss of the regular aforementioned calcium gradient in the epidermis. It has been hypothesized that impaired function of some TRP channels especially TRPC6 could be associated with the pathogenesis of atopic dermatitis. TRPC6 has been described as important mechanism of calcium entry in keratinocytes. Dysfunctional TRPC6 would lead to an impaired keratinocyte differentiation and thereby disrupt the epidermal barrier function. It has been shown that polymorphic variants of the Orai1 channels are associated with susceptibility towards atopic dermatitis.

One of the most characteristic symptoms of atopic dermatitis is severe itching. As the pruritus is not sufficiently alleviated by antihistamines, other mediators besides histamine are supposed to play an important role in this skin disease. Interleukin-31 as well as the neuro-peptide β-endorphin have been established as important mediators of itching in the atopic dermatitis. As mentioned above, IL-31 signaling is mediated via CRAC channels and leads to a release of β-endorphins. In this context, Orai and STIM molecules as well as TRPC6 are potential therapeutically targets in atopic dermatitis [2, 7-8, 11-13, 15, 17-18, 21-23, 25].

Psoriasis and Calcium

Psoriasis is clinically and histologically characterized by inflammation, hyper-proliferation and insufficient differentiation of keratinocytes. T-lymphocytes (TH1) play a crucial role in the inflammatory process of a psoriatic skin. Particularly, interferon-γ, TNF-α, Il-6 and Il-8 are proinflammatory cytokines in psoriasis. Recently Il-20 and IL-22 produced by T-cells as well as by keratinocytes were discussed as being responsible for altered differentiation of keratinocytes. As already described T-cell as well as keratinocyte activation, proliferation and differentiation strongly depend on calcium. In particular, functional CRAC channels are crucial for T-cell activation and their differentiation into effector T-cells. In cultured psoriatic keratinocytes, a down regulation of calcium influx and a defective calcium signaling was described. It has been reported that keratinocytes from psoriatic patients have lower endoplasmic reticulum calcium concentration and impaired CRAC channel function. Exactly these malfunctions have been considered as a cause for hyper-proliferation and insufficient differentiation. However, little is known about the role of the main molecular players STIM and ORAI in T-cells and keratinocytes of psoriatic patients. Nevertheless, these proteins could be an interesting potential target in treatment of psoriasis or of other inflammatory disorders. Besides the malfunctional Orai-STIM calcium entry pathway, a defect in TRP channel function was observed in psoriatic keratinocytes. In these cells, a down-regulation of TRPC6 channel expression and consequent impairment in differentiation and enhanced proliferation was observed.

Furthermore, the before described calcium gradient from low calcium at the basal layer to high calcium in the granular layer is disturbed in psoriatic skin and also has an impact on keratinocyte differentiation and leads to their hyper-proliferation. However, not much is known about the molecular identity of the factors responsible for the failure in the calcium gradient in the skin of psoriatic patients [2, 6-8, 11-12, 26-27].

Irritant Contact Dermatitis and Calcium

Irritant contact dermatitis is one of the most frequent skin diseases. In the essence of this disease are toxic compounds which produce a localized inflammation of the skin. During this inflammatory process, cytokines such as Interleukin-1-α, Il-6, Il-8, TNF-α, prostaglandins, ATP and endothelins are secreted by keratinocytes as well as by cells of the immune system. The increased local concentration of all these compounds further promotes the inflammation process.

Some of the most common strong irritants are substances such as Heptylamin, DMIPA, 2-4 Hexadienal, Piperazine, SLS, KOH and HCL while as weak irritants are substances known as sodium bisulphate, sodium bicarbonate, linalool axide and benzyl alcohol. A common feature of all these compounds is that they cause increase in the intracellular calcium concentration in keratinocytes. For example, heptylamine was shown to release calcium from the intracellular calcium stores thus having an indirect impact on the Orai channel function. Intracellular calcium measurements were even suggested as mean to evaluate irritant potential of a chemical [2, 8, 15, 28].

Conclusion

Calcium is an ubiquitous second messenger involved in a multitude of cellular events in virtually all human cells. As described above, skin cells as well as cells of the immune system cannot exhibit their physiological function without calcium. For the communication between the cells, calcium is also crucial. Inflammatory skin disease results from interplay of different cells types of the skin and the immune system. What is in the beginning usually meant as a mechanism of defense to some external factor, leads by defective, prolonged or exaggerated response of these cells to an inflammatory disorder. In this context, it is increasingly apparent that disturbed calcium signaling either in the local skin cells or/and the migrated immune cells play an important role in dermatitis. It is very important to note that not the sum of calcium signals appears to be defective in these skin diseases. The small changes in the dynamic, duration and kinetics of the calcium signals make the difference. New developments in the calcium research field bring more and more clarity in the calcium signaling machinery within the skin and also immune cells. Based on the initial findings described above, the future research on proteins such as Orai1-3 and STIM1-2 as well as the big family of TRP channels might yield better understanding on how calcium signals affect inflammatory skin diseases. These findings will hopefully be paralleled with development of novel activators or suppressors of these calcium channels, finally leading to development of novel therapeutics. Presently, however, the interplay of all these systems as well as the defects or changes that cause disease are far from fully elucidated.

References

[1] Bogeski I, Kappl R, Kummerow C, Gulaboski R, Hoth M, Niemeyer BA. Redox regulation of calcium ion channels: chemical and physiological aspects. *Cell Calcium.* 2011 Nov;50(5):407-23.

[2] Chang WC, Di Capite J, Singaravelu K, Nelson C, Halse V, Parekh AB. Local Ca2+ influx through Ca2+ release-activated Ca2+ (CRAC) channels stimulates production of an intracellular messenger and an intercellular pro-inflammatory signal. *J Biol Chem.* 2008 Feb 22;283(8):4622-31.

[3] Gwack Y, Feske S, Srikanth S, Hogan PG, Rao A. Signalling to transcription: store-operated Ca2+ entry and NFAT activation in lymphocytes. *Cell Calcium.* 2007 Aug;42(2):145-56.

[4] Parekh AB, Putney JW, Jr. Store-operated calcium channels. *Physiol Rev.* 2005 Apr;85(2):757-810.

[5] Pedersen SF, Owsianik G, Nilius B. TRP channels: an overview. *Cell Calcium.* 2005 Sep-Oct;38(3-4):233-52.

[6] Robert V, Triffaux E, Savignac M, Pelletier L. Calcium signalling in T-lymphocytes. *Biochimie.* 2011 Dec;93(12):2087-94.

[7] Beck B, Lehen'kyi V, Roudbaraki M, Flourakis M, Charveron M, Bordat P, et al. TRPC channels determine human keratinocyte differentiation: new insight into basal cell carcinoma. *Cell Calcium.* 2008 May;43 (5):492-505.

[8] Elias PM, Ahn SK, Denda M, Brown BE, Crumrine D, Kimutai LK, et al. Modulations in epidermal calcium regulate the expression of differentiation-specific markers. *J Invest Dermatol.* 2002 Nov;119 (5):1128-36.

[9] Fatherazi S, Belton CM, Izutsu KT. Sequential activation of store-operated currents in human gingival keratinocytes. *J Invest Dermatol.* 2003 Jul;121(1):120-31.

[10] Foggia L, Hovnanian A. Calcium pump disorders of the skin. *Am J Med Genet C Semin Med Genet. 2004* Nov 15;131C(1):20-31.

[11] Hancock GE, Kaplan G, Cohn ZA. Keratinocyte growth regulation by the products of immune cells. *J Exp Med.* 1988 Oct 1;168(4):1395-402.

[12] Hennings H, Holbrook KA. Calcium regulation of cell-cell contact and differentiation of epidermal cells in culture. An ultrastructural study. *Exp Cell Res.* 1983 Jan;143(1):127-42.

[13] Lee CH, Hong CH, Yu WT, Chuang HY, Huang SK, Chen GS, et al. Mechanistic correlations between two itch biomarkers, cytokine interleukin-31 and neuropeptide beta-endorphin, via STAT3/calcium axis in atopic dermatitis. *Br J Dermatol.* 2012 Oct;167(4):794-803.

[14] Pani B, Singh BB. Darier's disease: a calcium-signaling perspective. *Cell Mol Life Sci.* 2008 Jan;65(2):205-11.

[15] Proksch E, Folster-Holst R, Jensen JM. Skin barrier function, epidermal proliferation and differentiation in eczema. *J Dermatol Sci.* 2006 Sep;43(3):159-69.

[16] Savignac M, Edir A, Simon M, Hovnanian A. Darier disease : a disease model of impaired calcium homeostasis in the skin. *Biochim Biophys Acta.* 2011 May;1813(5):1111-7.

[17] Sun XD, You Y, Zhang L, Zheng S, Hong Y, Li J, et al. The possible role of TRPC6 in atopic dermatitis. *Med Hypotheses.* 2012 Jan;78(1):42-4.

[18] Woelfle U, Laszczyk MN, Kraus M, Leuner K, Kersten A, Simon-Haarhaus B, et al. Triterpenes promote keratinocyte differentiation in vitro, ex vivo and in vivo: a role for the transient receptor potential canonical (subtype) 6. *J Invest Dermatol.* 2010 Jan;130(1):113-23.

[19] Luger TA, Scholzen T, Brzoska T, Becher E, Slominski A, Paus R. Cutaneous immunomodulation and coordination of skin stress responses by alpha-melanocyte-stimulating hormone. *Ann N Y Acad Sci.* 1998 May 1;840:381-94.

[20] Stanisz H, Stark A, Kilch T, Schwarz EC, Muller CS, Peinelt C, et al. ORAI1 Ca(2+) channels control endothelin-1-induced mitogenesis and melanogenesis in primary human melanocytes. *J Invest Dermatol.* 2012 May;132(5):1443-51.

[21] Di Capite J, Parekh AB. CRAC channels and Ca2+ signaling in mast cells. *Immunol Rev.* 2009 Sep;231(1):45-58.

[22] Di Capite J, Shirley A, Nelson C, Bates G, Parekh AB. Intercellular Ca2+ wave propagation involving positive feedback between CRAC channels and cysteinyl leukotrienes. *FASEB J.* 2009 Mar;23(3):894-905.

[23] Gilfillan AM, Beaven MA. Regulation of mast cell responses in health and disease. *Crit Rev Immunol.* 2011;31(6):475-529.

[24] Cahalan MD, Chandy KG. The functional network of ion channels in T lymphocytes. *Immunol Rev.* 2009 Sep;231(1):59-87.

[25] Chang WC, Lee CH, Hirota T, Wang LF, Doi S, Miyatake A, et al. ORAI1 genetic polymorphisms associated with the susceptibility of atopic dermatitis in Japanese and Taiwanese populations. *PLoS One.* 2012;7(1):e29387.

[26] Leuner K, Kraus M, Woelfle U, Beschmann H, Harteneck C, Boehncke WH, et al. Reduced TRPC channel expression in psoriatic keratinocytes is associated with impaired differentiation and enhanced proliferation. *PLoS One.* 2011;6(2):e14716.

[27] Sabat R, Philipp S, Hoflich C, Kreutzer S, Wallace E, Asadullah K, et al. Immunopathogenesis of psoriasis. *Exp Dermatol.* 2007 Oct;16(10):779-98.

[28] Raoux M, Azorin N, Colomban C, Rivoire S, Merrot T, Delmas P, et al. Chemicals inducing acute irritant contact dermatitis mobilize intracellular calcium in human keratinocytes. *Toxicol In Vitro.* 2013 Feb;27(1):402-8.

In: Dermatitis
Editor: Cornelia Sigrid Lissi Müller
ISBN: 978-1-62618-997-3

Chapter IX

Treatment of Chronic Hand Eczema Using Orally Administered Alitretinoin

Claudia Pföhler [*] ***and Karin Braunert***
The Saarland University Hospital, Department of Dermatology,
Homburg/ Saar, Germany

Abstract

Treatment of chronic hand eczema (CHE) is a challenge for every dermatologist. With a one-year-prevalence of about 10% in Northern European Countries, CHE is a common disease. We conducted a prospective monocenter study to assess the efficacy and safety of orally administered alitretinoin in intensively pretreated patients with CHE refractory to topical corticosteroids.

Seventy patients (*m*=34, *f*=36) with severe CHE were enrolled in this clinical study. Median age was 52 years (*m*=50.5, range 25-71; *w*=54, range 25-72). Fifty-two patients showed hyperkeratotic CHE, nine dyshidrotic CHE and five other forms of CHE or CHE in combination with psoriasis pustulosa palmaris. Twenty-one out of 70 patients (30%) were smokers.

[*] Phone: 0049-6841-16-23840, Fax: 0049-6841-16 23845, Email: claudia.pfoehler@uks.eu and karin.braunert@ uks.eu.

Alitretinoin was administered orally in a daily dosage of 10 mg or 30 mg for at least 12 weeks. Response was defined as a clear reduction in Physician Global Assessment Score (PGAS) or in Total Lesion Symptom Score (TLSS).

Responses, defined as clear or almost clear hands, were achieved in 20 of 70 (28.6%) patients. This response rate is lower than in other clinical trials investigating the efficacy of alitretinoin in CHE. Median time to response in patients with clear or almost clear hands was 16 weeks (range 4-48 weeks). The mean grade of severity measured by PGAS was 3.37 before treatment and 1.78 after treatment. Treatment was generally well tolerated with dose-dependent adverse events. Twenty-two out of 70 patients (31.4%) showed no subjective side effects during treatment. Moderate side effects such as headache, mucocutaneous events such as dry lips or stomatitis, and laboratory abnormalities such as hyperlipidaemia or decreased levels of free thyroxine or thyroid-stimulating hormone were observed in 10/70 (14.2%) patients. We did not observe any severe adverse events.

In conclusion, the results of this monocenter study comply with results from other prospective trials using alitretinoin for the treatment of CHE, although the rate of patients with clear/almost clear hands was lower than described in other studies. Alitretinoin is a generally well-tolerated drug for the treatment of CHE that should be administered according to recently established treatment guidelines.

Introduction

Chronic hand eczema (CHE) is one of the most common inflammatory skin diseases. The one-year-prevalence in Northern European Countries is about 10% [1-2]. In certain jobs such as in health care workers the one-year-prevalence of CHE is approximately twofold higher with 21% [1]. Important risk factors for the development of hand eczema (HE) are female gender, the presence o contact allergy, atopy as well as wet work [1, 3]. In addition, HE belong to the most commonly reported occupational skin diseases [4]. The most common cause is contact dermatitis which may either result from irritant impacts or from contact allergy [4]. Nearly 80% of all occupational skin diseases, with the majority of them being HE, occur in seven groups with elevated risk to develop HE such as hairdressers, metal workers, health care workers, food industry workers, construction workers, cleaners, and painters [4]. It could be shown that in patients with occupational HE the prevalence of anxiety, depression and impaired health-related quality of life is very high [5].

In males, an association of severe HE with symptoms of anxiety and depression could be proved [5].

Until today, no generally accepted classification of HE exists [6]. There are classification schemes that characterize HE by its clinical presentation but sometimes it seems to be more reasonable to classify them by their underlying etiology [7-9]. The German guideline on the management of hand eczemas differentiates irritant or cumulative subtoxic HE, allergic HE, protein contact dermatitis and other HE forms (i.e. tylotic) according to their etiology [10]. Based on morphology, the guideline differentiates between dyshidrotic or vesicular HE, HE with erythema and scaling, hyperkeratotic-rhagadiform HE, and nummular eczema [10].

Treatment of HE first requires the elimination of causative factors. In case of contact allergy the causative allergens must be avoided, in case of irritation wet work must be reduced and adequate protection with protective ointments or gloves should be performed [11-12]. Topical treatment is mandatory for all patients. Effective emollients are needed and can be combined with topical corticosteroids, topical immunomodulators such as pimecrolimus or tacrolimus or topical photochemotherapy such as (cream)-PUVA [11-13]. In severe forms of HE a systemic therapy may be needed. Unfortunately, nearly all systemic drugs can only be used in an off-label setting [11-12]. This applies for oral corticosteroids, the oral retinoids acitretin or isotretinoin and immunosuppressants such as cyclosporine A, azathioprine or mycophenolate mofetil [11-12]. Furthermore, the pronounced toxicity of these substances limits their long-term use. Since a few years, oral alitretinoin is available for treatment of CHE [2, 11-12, 14-15]. The substance has been shown to be effective in all forms of HE [2]. Alitretinoin was effective in retreatment of relapsing HE and safety of use could be demonstrated even during extended treatment [11-12, 15]. The most frequent occurring adverse events under treatment with alitretinoin were headache, mucocutaneous events such as dry lips and skin or cheilitis or abnormalities in laboratory parameters such as elevated levels of cholesterol and triglycerids or reduced levels of thyroid-stimulating hormone (TSH) or thyroid hormones [2].

The aim of the study presented was to investigate the efficacy and safety of oral administered alitretinoin in CHE patients in a prospective monocenter study.

Table 1. Efficacy criteria: Physician Global Assessment (PGA)

PGA severity	Features	Intensity	Area involved
Severe	Erythema, scaling, hyperkeratosis, lichenification Vesiculation, oedema, pruritus or pain	At least one moderate or severe At least one severe	>30% of affected hand surface
Moderate	Erythema, scaling, hyperkeratosis, lichenification Vesiculation, oedema, pruritus or pain	At least one mild or moderate At least one moderate	10-30% of affected hand surface
Mild	Erythema, scaling, hyperkeratosis, lichenification Vesiculation, oedema, pruritus or pain	At least one mild At least one mild	< 10% of affected hand surface
Almost clear	Erythema, scaling, hyperkeratosis, lichenification Vesiculation, oedema, pruritus or pain	At least one mild Absent	< 10% of affected hand surface
Clear	Erythema, scaling, hyperkeratosis, lichenification Vesiculation, oedema, pruritus or pain	Absent Absent	Absent

Material and Methods

Patients

Seventy patients (m=34, f=36) with severe CHE were enrolled in this clinical study. Median age was 52 years (m=50.5, range 25-71; f=54, range 25-

72). Fifty-two patients showed hyperkeratotic CHE, nine dyshidrotic CHE and five other forms of CHE or CHE in combination with psoriasis pustulosa palmaris. Twenty-one out of 70 patients (30%) were smokers. Patients suffered from CHE for at least 6 months or longer and had been refractory to a treatment with potent topical corticosteroids. All patients had received standard skin care including topical emollients and had avoided allergens or irritants without significant improvement. Earlier systemic treatment for CHE was no exclusion criterion, but a wash out period of at least 14 days was mandatory.

Treatment

All patients received either 10mg or 30 mg alitretinoin daily for at least 12 weeks. Topical therapy including emollients, topical steroids, tar preaparations or calcineurin inhibitors was allowed. Orally administered antihistamines to treat pruritic forms of CHE were allowed too.

Evaluation Instruments

Severity of HE was defined according to the Physicial Global Assessment (PGA) (Table 1) and the severity of each symptom was described with the modified Total Lesion Symptom Score (mTLSS) (Tabel 2). Photos were taken at the beginning of oral treatment with alitretinoin and periodically afterwards. Laboratory investigation included standard hematology, fasting blood chemistry and thyroid function. Adverse events (AE) were recorded throughout therapy and during follow-up. Classification and grading of AE was performed using Common Terminology Criteria for Adverse Events (CTCAE).

Results

Responses, defined as clear or almost clear hands, were achieved in 20 of 70 (28.6%) patients (Figure 1). Median time to response in patients with clear or almost clear hands was 16 weeks (range 4-48 weeks). The mean grade of severity measured by PGAS was 3.37 before treatment and 1.78 after treatment. Dose-dependent efficacy was observed for all types of CHE with hyperkeratotic HE forms showing the highest response rate (19/52 patients; 36.5 %). Treatment was generally well tolerated with dose-dependent adverse events. Twenty-two out of 70 patients (31.4%) showed no subjective side effects during treatment. Moderate side effects such as headache, mucocutaneous events such as dry lips or stomatitis, and laboratory abnormalities such as hyperlipidaemia or decreased levels of free thyroxine or thyroid-stimulating hormone were observed in 10/70 (14.27%) patients. We did not observe any severe adverse events.

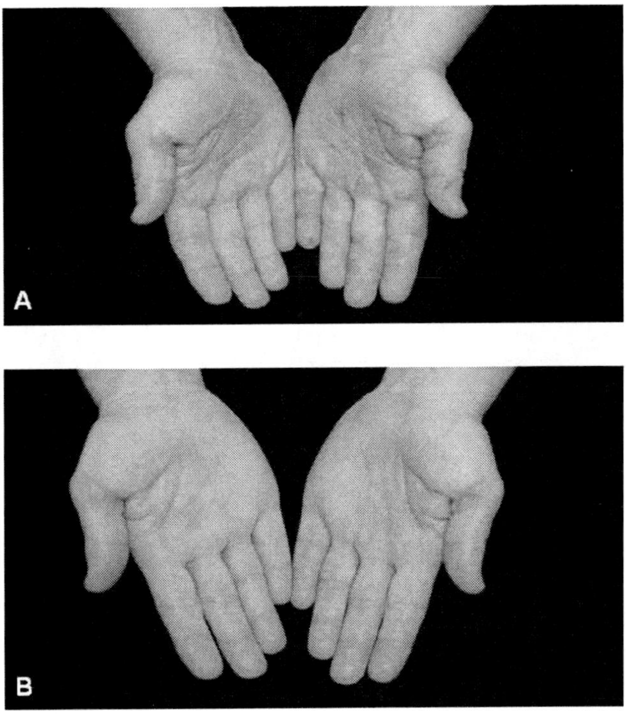

Figure 1. 47-year old female patient with hyperkeratotic CHE; at baseline (A) and after treatment with alitretinoin administered orally in a daily dose of 30 mg for four months (B).

Conclusion

In general, the results of this monocenter study using orally administered alitretinoin in patients with CHE refractory to topical corticosteroid treatment are consistent with those of previously published controlled and uncontrolled trials [2, 11-12, 15]. However, responses, defined as clear or almost clear hands, were only achieved in less than 30% of our patients. This response rate is lower than in other clinical trials investigating the efficacy of alitretinoin in CHE. In the BACH study responses were achieved in 48%, in the TOCCATA study in 56.7% [2, 10]. Even an opel-label study including CHE patients who did not fully respond to alitretinoin treatment in the BACH study showed higher response rates of 50 % in the 30mg group and 39% in the 10mg group [15]. Possibly, the high percentage of smokers (30%) in our study collective has played an important role for our lower response rates. Smoking, especially excessive consumption of more than 15 cigarettes per day has been shown to be associated with the prevalence of HE and with severity of disease [16-17]. However, as in other studies performed before, alitretinoin was effective in both dosing regimens, but the 30 mg dose lead to higher response rates and more rapid responses.

No adverse events were reported in 31.4%. Moderate side effects such as headache, mucocutaneous events such as dry lips or stomatitis, and laboratory abnormalities such as hyperlipidaemia or decreased levels of free thyroxine or thyroid-stimulating hormone were observed in 14.2% patients. We did not observe any severe adverse events. No adverse events lead to discontinuation of therapy. Hence, the rate of AEs in our study was considerably lower than for instance in the BACH study (20%) or the TOCCATA study (23%) [2, 10]. However, we are aware of the limits of our study. The most important things with influence on our study results are the monocenter design and the fact that the use of potent topical therapies was allowed.

However, the results of this monocenter study emphasize the results of other studies investigating the efficacy and safety of orally administered alitretinoin in patients with CHE refractory to topical treatment with potent corticosteroids. Guidelines on the management of HE recommend the use of alitretinoin in moderate to severe forms of HE, especially in cases in which previous treatment with corticosteroids, topical calcineurininhibitors or phototherapy such as cream-PUVA therapy had failed [14]. Alitretinoin is a usally well-tolerated and safe substance with a very short half-life time in comparison to isotretinoin or acitretin [18]. However, alitretinoin belongs to the retinoic acids and is a teratogen substance. In female patients with child-bearing potential safety instructions and an effective contraception are therefore mandatory. This may limit the use of alitretinoin in a subgroup of CHE patients.

Table 2. Efficacy criteria: modified Total Lesion Symptom Score (mTLSS)

Parameter	Description of severity
Erythema	0 = absent 1 = faint erythema 2 = prominent redness 3 = deep intense red color
Scaling	0 = absent 1 = Slight flaking over limited areas, mostly fine scales 2 = Flaking over widespread area(s), coarser scales 3 = Desquamation >30% of the hand with coarse thick scales
Lichenification/ hyperkeratosis	0 = absent 1 = mild thickening with exaggerated skin lines over limited areas 2 = palpable thickening over widespread area(s) 3 = prominent thickening over widespread area(s) with exaggeration of normal skin markings
Vesiculation	0 = absent 1 = scattered vesicules affecting up to 10% of hand, no erosion 2 = scattered or clustered vesicules affecting up to 30% of hand, no erosion or excoriation 3 = high densitiy of vesicules over large area(s) <u>or</u> with erosion or excoriation
Oedema	0 = absent 1 = dermal swelling over less than 10% of hands 2 = definite dermal swelling with skin induration over widespread area(s) 3 = dermal swelling with skin induration over widespread area(s)
Fissures	0 = absent 1 = cracked skin affecting a small area of hand 2 = one or more deep fissures and causing pain 3 = one or more deep fissures and causing bleeding or severe pain
Pruritus/pain	0 = absent 1 = occasional, slight discomfort a few times per day 2 = intermittent, causing discomfort frequently during the day 3 = persistent or interfering with sleep

In conclusion, alitretinoin is the first systemic drug that has been approved for treatment of HE. The advantage of alitretinoin over other systemic drugs such as corticosteroids, cyclosporine A, azathioprine or mycophenolate mofetil is that it has no immunosuppressive effects and evokes no rebound-effect after treatment is stopped. Therefore, alitretinoin has become a valuable treatment option in patients with a high disease burden and few therapeutic options.

References

[1] Ibler KS, Jemec GB, Flyvholm MA, Diepgen TL, Jensen A, Agner T. Hand eczema: prevalence and risk factors of hand eczema in a population of 2274 healthcare workers. *Contact Dermatitis.* 2012 Oct;67(4):200-7.

[2] Ruzicka T, Lynde CW, Jemec GB, Diepgen T, Berth-Jones J, Coenraads PJ, et al. Efficacy and safety of oral alitretinoin (9-cis retinoic acid) in patients with severe chronic hand eczema refractory to topical corticosteroids: results of a randomized, double-blind, placebo-controlled, multicentre trial. *Br J Dermatol.* 2008 Apr;158(4):808-17.

[3] Apfelbacher CJ, Akst W, Molin S, Schmitt J, Bauer A, Weisshaar E, et al. CARPE: a registry project of the German Dermatological Society (DDG) for the characterization and care of chronic hand eczema. *J Dtsch Dermatol Ges.* 2011 Sep;9(9):682-8.

[4] Diepgen TL. Occupational skin diseases. *J Dtsch Dermatol Ges.* 2012 May;10(5):297-313; quiz 4-5.

[5] Boehm D, Schmid-Ott G, Finkeldey F, John SM, Dwinger C, Werfel T, et al. Anxiety, depression and impaired health-related quality of life in patients with occupational hand eczema. *Contact Dermatitis.* 2012 Oct;67(4):184-92.

[6] Johansen JD, Hald M, Andersen BL, Laurberg G, Danielsen A, Avnstorp C, et al. Classification of hand eczema: clinical and aetiological types. Based on the guideline of the Danish Contact Dermatitis Group. *Contact Dermatitis.* 2011 Jul;65(1):13-21.

[7] Cronin E. Clinical patterns of hand eczema in women. *Contact Dermatitis.* 1985 Sep;13(3):153-61.

[8] Goetzsche PC. Rational Diagnosis and Treatment, Evidence-Based Clinical Decision-Making. 4th ed. Chichester: John Wiley & Sons; 2008.

[9] Wilkinson ds. *Introduction, definition and classification.* 1st ed. Mennè TM, H.I., editor: Boca Raton, FL, Ann Arbor, MI, London; 1994.

[10] Diepgen TL, Elsner P, Schliemann S, Fartasch M, Kollner A, Skudlik C, et al. Guideline on the management of hand eczema ICD-10 Code: L20. L23. L24. L25. L30. *J Dtsch Dermatol Ges*. 2009 May;7 Suppl 3:S1-16.

[11] Bissonnette R, Diepgen TL, Elsner P, English J, Graham-Brown R, Homey B, et al. Redefining treatment options in chronic hand eczema (CHE). *J Eur Acad Dermatol Venereol.* 2010 May;24 Suppl 3:1-20.

[12] Bissonnette R, Worm M, Gerlach B, Guenther L, Cambazard F, Ruzicka T, et al. Successful retreatment with alitretinoin in patients with relapsed chronic hand eczema. *Br J Dermatol.* 2010 Feb 1;162(2):420-6.

[13] van Gils RF, Boot CR, Knol DL, Rustemeyer T, van Mechelen W, van der Valk PG, et al. The effectiveness of integrated care for patients with hand eczema: results of a randomized, controlled trial. *Contact Dermatitis.* 2012 Apr;66(4):197-204.

[14] Diepgen TL, Pfarr E, Zimmermann T. Efficacy and tolerability of alitretinoin for chronic hand eczema under daily practice conditions: results of the TOCCATA open study comprising 680 patients. *Acta Derm Venereol.* 2012 May;92(3):251-5.

[15] Lynde C, Cambazard F, Ruzicka T, Sebastian M, Brown TC, Maares J. Extended treatment with oral alitretinoin for patients with chronic hand eczema not fully responding to initial treatment. *Clin Exp Dermatol.* 2012 Oct;37(7):712-7.

[16] Anveden Berglind I, Alderling M, Meding B. Life-style factors and hand eczema. *Br J Dermatol.* 2011 Sep;165(3):568-75.

[17] Meding B, Alderling M, Wrangsjo K. Tobacco smoking and hand eczema: a population-based study. *Br J Dermatol.* 2010 Oct;163(4):752-6.

[18] Schmitt-Hoffmann AH, Roos B, Sauer J, Spickermann J, Stoeckel K, Edwards D, et al. Pharmacokinetics, efficacy and safety of alitretinoin in moderate or severe chronic hand eczema. *Clin Exp Dermatol.* 2011 Apr;36 Suppl 2:29-34.

In: Dermatitis
Editor: Cornelia Sigrid Lissi Müller
ISBN: 978-1-62618-997-3

Chapter X

Topical Anti-inflammatory Treatment

Mylène Niclou[*]
The Saarland University Hospital,
Department of Dermatology, Homburg/Saar, Germany

Abstract

Nowadays a large variety of systemic medications, which have appeared over recent decades, have improved the treatment possibilities for many skin diseases, but topical treatment is still one of the most important therapy options in dermatology, and is particularly indispensable for inflammatory disorders. Of the topical medications, glucocorticoids are still the most important and most-widely prescribed. Today, however, immunosuppressant and immunomodulatory drugs from the macrolide group such as tacrolimus and pimecrolimus (the so-called calcineurin inhibitors) provide an alternative to glucocorticoids and have an important role to play in local anti-inflammatory therapy. The use of topical glucocorticoids or calcineurin inhibitors is not only important in acute flares but recently the concept of proactive therapy has become more and more popular in topical treatment of skin diseases such as for example atopic eczema.

[*] Phone: 0049-6841-16-23966. Fax: 0049-6841-16 23845. Email: mylene.niclou@uks.eu.

Introduction

Nowadays a large variety of systemic medications, which have appeared over recent decades, have improved the treatment possibilities for many skin diseases, but topical treatment is still one of the most important therapy options in dermatology, and is particularly indispensable for inflammatory disorders. Of the topical medications, glucocorticoids are still the most important and most-widely prescribed. Today, however, immunosuppressant and immunomodulatory drugs from the macrolide group such as tacrolimus and pimecrolimus (the so-called calcineurin inhibitors) provide an alternative to glucocorticoids and have an important role to play in local anti-inflammatory therapy. The use of topical glucocorticoids or calcineurin inhibitors is not only important in acute flares but recently the concept of proactive therapy has become more and more popular in topical treatment of skin diseases such as for example atopic eczema.

Glucocorticoids

In exacerbation management of inflammatory skin diseases the use of anti-inflammatory treatment based on topical glucocorticosteroids and topical calcineurin inhibitors is indispensable. Of the topical medications, glucocorticoids are still the most important and most-widely prescribed. They are the first-line anti-inflammatory treatment and they all originate from one chemical structure. Cortisol and cortisone are the physiological equivalents; they are produced in a circadian rhythm in the suprarenal glands and obey a strict control system that involves the hypothalamus and the anterior pituitary. The production maximum is in the early morning, the minimum around midnight. Cortisone treatment can be administrated systemically or topically. The physiological glucocorticoids must be distinguished from their synthetic derivatives, but their working mechanism is similar. Glucocorticoids bind to the intercellular-located glucocorticoid receptor. Whilst unligated the receptor is bound to a large complex of heat shock proteins. The binding provokes a configuration changement of the receptor and dissociation from the heat shock proteins. The free receptor then translocates from the cytoplasma to the cell core, where it provokes a changing of the transcription rate of the glucocorticoid-sensitive genes which influences the production of proteins [1]. Substances like arachidonic acid, prostaglandin, leukotrien, thromboxane, platelet activating factor, TNF-alpha, IL-1, IL-2, IL-6 and plasminogen activator are inhibited, T-cell-activity is slowed down, the apoptosis of eosinophils is induced and the membranes of neutrophils are stabilised. This working mechanism explains why the main therapy effects appear not immediately after treatment but in general after a few hours.

To improve the reaction time and efficiency of the therapy halogenated versions of the synthetic derivates were developed (with fluoride or chloride added to the chemical structure in position 6α, 9α or 16α) [1]. Unfortunately this process does not just improve the working mechanism, but also increases the incidence of possible side effects. This is why esterification of the synthetic derivates was developed for topical treatment: esterification increases the lipophilia and improves the skin penetration effect, with reduced side effects [2]. Additional methods of modifying the effect of topical glucocorticoids include changing the choice of the base, adding urea to the base and different forms of application (for example occlusive bandages or wet wraps can increase the effect).

Topical glucocorticoids are grouped by potency in 4 categories and nowadays a wide variety of substances are available, the most potent one being Clobetasolpropionat.

Topical glucocorticoids should always be chosen according to a risk-benefit ratio, and the choice should take into account the age of the patient, the area that needs treatment (for example the face, the genitals, the axilla and the inguinal fold should always be treated with a less potent glucocorticoid than the rest of the body), and the gender (possible pregnancy should be considered). Glucocorticoids are applied to inflamed skin according to the needs of the skin [3]. To benefit from the therapy it is essential that the application is carried out correctly and as prescribed, therefore the instruction of the patient is of great importance. If carried out correctly one application daily can be sufficient [4-5].

The possible side effects after a topical application of glucocorticoids are numerous, therefore prescription should only be made by doctors with appropriate experience and their use should always be considered critically. Possible local side effects include epidermal atrophy and the thinning-out of the epidermis, hypertrichosis, steroid acne, atrophy and thinning-out of the connective tissue, striae distensae, disorder of pigmentation, stippled skin, teleangiectasias, steroid purpura, perioral dermatitis, slowing down of wound healings and weakening of the immune system [2]. Very rarely a contact allergy can appear (although usually the allergy is caused by other ingredients of the topical treatment: a contact allergy to glucocorticoids is not very common). The possibility of systemic side effects should never be forgotten: they can appear after a long topical treatment or sometimes in children if the therapy was not adjusted to their age. They include for example cushing syndrome, depression of the adrenal function, hypopotassemia, osteoporosis, diabetes mellitus and glaucoma [2]. In addition the rebound effect can cause problems and frustration in patients, therefore a long topical treatment with glucocorticoids should always be reduced gradually.

Calcineurin Inhibitors

Ciclosporin A originates from the macrolide group. In the early eighties it revolutionised the therapy of patients after organ transplantation [1]. Since the nineties cyclosporine A has been used as a systemic drug in the therapy of psoriasis and in severe forms of atopic eczema. Applied topically the effect is very small (probably the big molecular size prevents a proper penetration through the skin), therefore tacrolimus and pimecrolimus, both members of the macrolide group with a smaller molecular size, are used in the topical anti-inflammatory treatment [2]. Tacrolimus is produced by the fungus *Streptomyces tsukubaensis* (the name originates from tsukubaensis macrolide immunosuppressive) and pimecrolimus is produced by *Streptomyces hygroscopicus*.

For both drugs the working mechanism is similar and comparable to the effect of cyclosporine A. By blocking calcineurin the production of interleukin 2 is blocked and T-cell activity is reduced. Inside the cell tacrolimus for example forms a complex with the FK 506 binding protein which then blocks calcineurin. Calcineurin is a phosphatase that dephosphorylates a transcription factor (NF-ATc, nuclear factor of activated T-cells) in activated T-cells which in turn provokes the production of pro-inflammatory zytokines (such as interleukin 2 and other TH-1-zytokines) [2]. Interleukin 2 plays an important role in the proliferation of lymphozytes. The working mechanism of calcineurin inhibitors explains their anti-inflammatory effect: they have a slowing down effect on cell proliferation.

Tacrolimus and pimecrolimus are used as second line anti-inflammatory therapy in adults and children over 2 years for the neck and face, and for patients who do not respond to or cannot tolerate topical glucocorticoid. They should not be used in pregnancy and whilst breast-feeding. In general they are used to treat atopic eczema; there are a lot of clinical trials demonstrating the efficiency and safety of the treatment of atopic eczema with calcineurin inhibitors. However, the treatment should not be continuous, but should only be intermittent and for a short period and it should be ended as soon as the symptoms have disappeared. Other inflammatory skin diseases (for example lichen planus, granuloma anulare, etc...) can be treated with the off-label use of calcineurin inhibitors. A very important advantage of tacrolimus and pimecrolimus is that they do not cause skin atrophy, which explains why their use is preferred for sensitive body areas such as the face, the genitals, the axilla and the inguinal fold. In fact they can be used on any part of the body apart from the mucosa and erosive lesions. Treatment should commence as soon as symptoms appear.

Patients should be advised that in the first days following application a transient warmth sensation and/or an itching or burning of the treated skin can occur. It can start after a few minutes and last for more than an hour. In general this side effect disappears after a few days of treatment [6-7]. As there is not a great deal of experience of the application of tacrolimus and pimecrolimus with occlusive bandages, this method of application should be avoided as there may be a risk of increased systemic absorption [3]. Another side effect that is discussed from time to time is a potential increased risk of lymphoma and white skin cancer after long-term use. In a very small number of cases (less than 1 percent) the patients suffered from swollen lymph nodes during the topical treatment (which in almost all the cases was due to a secondary infection of, for example, the teeth or the respiratory system) and if this occurs the cause should always be investigated. However, with chronic eczemas, an elevated risk of lymphoma is discussed in any event, and as the levels of tacrolimus and pimecrolimus in the blood of patients undergoing topical treatment with these calcineurin inhibitors are low, there is no obvious link and to the present day there is no scientific evidence of an increased risk for the development of such a malignancy. However, as it is known the systemic administration of cyclosporine increases the photocarcinogenicity risk, an effective UV protection is recommended whilst using topical calcineurin inhibitors (for example avoiding the sun, using sunscreens etc) [8]. In addition calcineurin inhibitors should not be applied to an area of the skin where there is a potential malignancy or pre-malignancy. Nor should they be applied to the area of a viral skin infection, such as herpes simplex or chicken pox, as the immunosuppressive effect of the treatment exacerbates the viral infection. This same effect creates a small increase in the risk of the patient suffering an outbreak of an existing but latent viral skin infection: generalised viral infections such as eczema herpeticatum and eczema molluscatum have been observed during topical calcineurin inhibator treatment [9-10]. Finally, calcineurin inhibitors should not be used with patients that either were born with an immunodeficiency or are undergoing immunosuppressive therapy.

Proactive Therapy

The use of topical glucocorticoids or calcineurin inhibitors is not only important in acute flares but recently the concept of the proactive therapy has become more and more popular in the topical treatment of skin diseases such as for example atopic eczema, with the aim of preventing the eczema reappearing or at least reducing the frequency, duration or severity of a flare-up. The concept is of a low-dose and long-term anti-inflammatory treatment.

In proactive therapy the treatment, which could have either gluco-corticoids or calcineurin inhibitors as the active ingredient, is used not every day but usually two times a week once per day usually on the parts of the body that are most often the site of the flare-up, whilst the rest of the body should be treated by emollients [3]. If the treatment is with calcineurin inhibitors, then after not more than twelve months the therapy should be critically reviewed as at present there are no studies of the results of treatments lasting longer than this period. If the treatment is with glucocorticoids, then care must be taken to watch out for the typical long term side effects of their topical application such as skin atrophy. When looking at the working mechanisms of glucocorticoids and calcineurin inhibitors it may seem worthwhile to combine both drugs to achieve better treatment results but in 2010 Meurer et al. showed that the combination of topical corticosteroids with topical calcineurin inhibitors does not seem to be useful, at least in patients with a severe atopic eczema. The safety profile and the efficacy of 1% pimecrolimus cream combined with fluticasone were similar to that of flucticasone alone [11].

References

[1] Karow T. Allgemeine und spezielle Pharamakologie: Selbstverlag; 2007.

[2] Plewig GL, M., Burgdorf W., Hertl, M., Ruzicka, T. Braun- Falco's Dermatologie Venerologie und Allergologie: Springer Verlag; 2012.

[3] Ring J, Alomar A, Bieber T, Deleuran M, Fink-Wagner A, Gelmetti C, et al. Guidelines for treatment of atopic eczema (atopic dermatitis) Part II. *J Eur Acad Dermatol Venereol.* 2012 Sep;26(9):1176-93.

[4] Charman C, Williams H. The use of corticosteroids and corticosteroid phobia in atopic dermatitis. *Clin Dermatol.* 2003 May-Jun;21(3):193-200.

[5] Queille C, Pommarede R, Saurat JH. Efficacy versus systemic effects of six topical steroids in the treatment of atopic dermatitis of childhood. *Pediatr Dermatol.* 1984 Jan;1(3):246-53.

[6] Chen SL, Yan J, Wang FS. Two topical calcineurin inhibitors for the treatment of atopic dermatitis in pediatric patients: a meta-analysis of randomized clinical trials. *J Dermatolog Treat.* 2010 May;21(3):144-56.

[7] Ruzicka T, Bieber T, Schopf E, Rubins A, Dobozy A, Bos JD, et al. A short-term trial of tacrolimus ointment for atopic dermatitis. European Tacrolimus Multicenter Atopic Dermatitis Study Group. *N Engl J Med.* 1997 Sep 18;337(12):816-21.

[8] Reitamo S, Van Leent EJ, Ho V, Harper J, Ruzicka T, Kalimo K, et al. Efficacy and safety of tacrolimus ointment compared with that of hydrocortisone acetate ointment in children with atopic dermatitis. *J Allergy Clin Immunol.* 2002 Mar;109(3):539-46.

[9] Lubbe J, Pournaras CC, Saurat JH. Eczema herpeticum during treatment of atopic dermatitis with 0.1% tacrolimus ointment. *Dermatology.* 2000;201(3):249-51.

[10] Wetzel S, Wollenberg A. Eczema molluscatum in tacrolimus treated atopic dermatitis. Eur J Dermatol. 2004 Jan-Feb;14(1):73-4.

[11] Meurer M, Eichenfield LF, Ho V, Potter PC, Werfel T, Hultsch T. Addition of pimecrolimus cream 1% to a topical corticosteroid treatment regimen in paediatric patients with severe atopic dermatitis: a randomized, double-blind trial. *J Dermatolog Treat.* 2010 May;21 (3):157-66.

In: Dermatitis
Editor: Cornelia Sigrid Lissi Müller
ISBN: 978-1-62618-997-3

Chapter XI

1,25-Dihydroxyvitamin D3 and Analogues in the Treatment of Psoriasis and Other Skin Conditions

Jörg Reichrath [*]
The Saarland University Hospital, Department of Dermatology, Homburg/ Saar, Germany

Abstract

The skin is a tissue that produces and represents a target tissue for vitamin D compounds. The epidermal synthesis of 1,25(OH)2D3 is of high importance because 1,25(OH)2D3 regulates key cellular functions in keratinocytes and dermal immunocompetent cells. Because of their antiproliferative and differentiation-inducing effects 1,25(OH)2D3 and other vitamin D compounds are very efficient in the treatment of the skin disease psoriasis. In addition, the known therapeutical effect of UVB-light-therapy in the topical psoriasis could, at least partially, include the UVB-induced synthesis of 1,25(OH)2D3. Recent findings related to the cutaneous metabolism of vitamin D compounds may result in new concepts for therapeutical applications of vitamin D compounds in skin diseases.

[*] Phone: 0049-6841-16-23802, Fax: 0049-6841-16 23845, Email: joerg.reichrath@uks.eu.

Introduction

Vitamin D is photochemically produced by UV-B action in the skin [1,2]. Interestingly, the skin represents not exclusively the site of vitamin D production, but is also an important target tissue for the biologically active vitamin D metabolite 1,25(OH)2D3 (1,25-dihydroxyvitamin D3, calcitriol), a seco-steroid hormone [3,4]. 1,25(OH)2D3 acts via both genomic and non-genomic effects. Non-genomic effects of 1,25(OH)2D3 and analogues are at least in part related to effects on intracellular calcium 5,6. In various skin cells including keratinocytes and in other cell types, 1,25(OH)2D3 increases rapidly free cytosolic calcium levels [5,6]. Genomic effects of 1,25(OH)2D3 are the result of binding to the vitamin D receptor (VDR), a nuclear receptor protein that is present in target tissues and binds 1,25(OH)2D3 calcitriol with high affinity (KD 10-9 - 10-10 M) and low capacity [7,8]. When the human VDR was cloned 9 , sequence analysis revealed that this protein belongs to the superfamily of trans-acting transcriptional regulatory factors, which includes the steroid and thyroid hormone receptors and the retinoic acid receptors [9]. Binding of 1,25(OH)2D3 to VDR results in the phosphorylation of the receptor complex that, as a consequence, activates the transcription of 1,25(OH)2D3-sensitive target genes, including genes involved in cellular differentiation and proliferation. VDR depends on auxillary factors for sufficient DNA-binding [10]. These auxillary proteins include the retinoid-X receptors (RXR-α,-β,-γ) that were demonstrated to heterodimerize with VDR, thus both increasing the transcriptional function and DNA binding to vitamin D response elements (VDRE) in the promotor region of target genes [10,11]. In the human skin, both VDR and RXR-α are expressed in many cell types, including keratinocytes, fibroblasts, Langerhans cells, sebaceous gland cells, endothelial cells and most cell types related to the skin immune system [12,13].

In vitro studies demonstrated that 1,25(OH)2D3 is very effective in inducing the terminal differentiation and in inhibiting the proliferation of cultured human keratinocytes in a dose-dependent manner [14-16]. Moreover, 1,25(OH)2D3 exerts potent effects on many cell types involved in immunologic reactions, including lymphocytes, macrophages and Langerhans cells [17,18].

The effects of 1,25(OH)2D3 on the melanin pigmentation system are still controversely discussed, but most studies do not support the possibility that calcitriol might regulate melanogenesis in human skin [19].

Psoriasis: Pathogenesis, Immunology, and Histology Of skin Lesions

Psoriasis is a chronic skin disease of unknown etiology characterized by hyperproliferation and inflammation of the skin. It may affect the skin, nails and joints in 1%-3% of the world's population with severe impacts on quality of life. Several different types of psoriasis can be diagnosed, with psoriasis vulgaris (plaque psoriasis) being the most common form. Psoriasis vulgaris is characterized by sharply demarcated, raised, inflamed, red lesions (plaques) covered by silvery white scales. The peak age of onset for this disease is the second decade, but psoriasis may first appear at any age from infancy to the aged [20]. Population, family and twin studies showed a strong but very complex genetic component that underlies the development of psoriatic skin lesions [21]. Psoriasis has long been known to be associated with certain HLA antigens, including HLA-Cw6, although there is no proof that a psoriasis susceptibility gene exists at this locus [22]. Many studies support the hypothesis that epidermal hyperproliferation in psoriasis may be caused by cells of the immune system, most likely T- lymphocytes [23]. Activated T-cells present in psoriatic lesions express HLA-DR, the interleukin-2 receptor (CD 25) and secrete specific immune mediators and cytokines, including IL-2 and interferon-γ [24-26]. Therefore, psoriasis vulgaris represents a so called Th1 profile disease (characterized by T-lymphocyte secretion of IL-2, IL-12, and interferon-γ) [27]. In contrast, atopic dermatitis represents a so called Th2 profile skin disease, that is characterized by T-cell secretion of IL-4, IL-5 and IL-10 [28]. The disease-triggering activation signal for the development of psoriatic lesions is still unknown, however there is increasing evidence that superantigens such as the N-terminal component of bacterial M-proteins may be of importance for the initiation of T-cell proliferation in psoriasis [29]. On the other hand, the hypothesis that immune cells may represent the primarily affected cell type in psoriasis has been challenged again when it was shown in adult mice that inducible epidermal deletion of Jun proteins result in psoriasis-like skin disease and arthritis [30].

Histological examination reveals in general, epidermal hyperplasia, in which the granular layer may be lost and the stratum corneum shows parakeratosis can be found. Typical lesions histologically demonstrate elongation of the dermal papillae, with a relatively thin epidermis at the top of the papillae. Epidermis may demonstrate infiltration with T-lymphocytes and/or neutrophiles, that can extend into spongiform pustules of Kogoj or Munro microabscesses [31].

Clinical Investigations of Vitamin D compounds in Psoriasis and Other Skin Diseases

1,25(OH)2D3 and Analogues for Treatment of Psoriasis

The use of 1,25(OH)2D3 and analogues for treatment of psoriasis resulted from two different lines of investigation. Before launching clinical trials in 1985, MacLaughlin and associates demonstrated that psoriatic fibroblasts are partially resistant to the antiproliferative effects of 1,25(OH)2D3 [32]. The other line of investigation resulted from a clinical observation reported in 1985 by Morimoto and Kumahara. They demonstrated that a patient, who was treated orally with 1α-hydroxyvitamin D3 for osteoporosis, had a dramatic remission of his psoriasis [33].

Morimoto et al. reported a follow up study, showing that almost 80% of 17 patients with psoriasis who were treated orally with 1α-hydroxyvitamin D3 (1,0 ug/day for up to 6 month) showed clinically significant improvement [35].

It has been shown that many different vitamin D compounds, including calcitriol, calcipotriol, tacalcitol, maxacalcitol and beocalcidiol are effective and safe in the topical treatment of psoriasis [35-39]. Topical 1,25(OH)2D3 is very effective and safe in the long term treatment of psoriasis [40]. After topical therapy for 6-8 weeks in clinical trials, calcipotriol ointment and cream reduced mean PASI (Psoriasis Area and Severity Index) scores by 55-72% and 49-50%, respectively [41]. Applied twice daily topically (50 μg/g ointment) per week, calcipotriol, the synthetic analogue of 1,25(OH)2D3 was shown to be slightly more effective in the topical treatment of psoriasis than betametasone 17-valerate ointment [42]. Calcipotriol cream has been reported to be more cosmetically acceptable than coal tar in a small trial in patients with psoriasis [43]. Calcipotriol ointment was compared with short-contact dithranol cream therapy [44]. At the end of treatment, no statistically significant differences were found between the calcipotriol and the dithranol group. In a large, randomized, double-blind, controlled trial, twice-daily calcipotriol cream was significantly more effective than once-daily calcipotriol cream [45].

A randomized, multicenter comparison of the efficacy and safety of twice daily applications of 1,25(OH)2D3 3 microg/g ointment vs. calcipotriol [50] microg/g ointment in subjects with mild to moderate chronic plaque-type psoriasis has been reported [46]. Efficacy evaluations comprised global improvement (on a 4-point scale from 0: no change or worse, to 3: clear or almost clear) assessed by both the investigator and the subject. Efficacy also included the 'dermatological sum score' at each study visit. Safety evaluations included adverse event reporting, cutaneous safety assessed by the clinical investigator and cutaneous discomfort assessment by the subject (both on a 5-point scale from 0: none, to 4: very severe). were recruited. At week 12, the LSmean score of global improvement rated by the investigator was 2.27 for 1,25(OH)2D3 and 2.22 for calcipotriol. This difference was not statistically significant, with 1,25(OH)2D3 showing to be non-inferior to calcipotriol for global improvement. This same parameter was scored by the subject, with a mean of 2.12 for 1,25(OH)2D3 and 2.09 for calcipotriol. The percentage of patients with at least marked improvement tended to be in favour of 1,25(OH)2D3 (95.7% vs. 85% for calcipotriol). However, differences were not statistically significant. The mean worst score for the cutaneous safety assessment was higher in the calcipotriol group (0.3 vs. 0.1 and 0.4 vs. 0.2, by the investigator and the patient, respectively). These differences were statistically significant in favour of a better safety profile for 1,25(OH)2D3 (P=0.0035). Fourteen dermatological and treatment-related adverse events were reported with calcipotriol vs. only five with 1,25(OH)2D3 for a total of 22 adverse events reported throughout the study. The authors concluded that 1,25(OH)2D3 administered twice daily over a 12-week treatment period demonstrated similar efficacy as compared to calcipotriol, while showing a significantly better safety profile. It has been reported that a mild dermatitis can be seen in about 10% of patients treated with calcipotriol (50 μg/g), particularly on the face [47]. This side effect (mild dermatitis on the face) is not reported after topical treatment with calcitriol.

A multicentre study, analyzing the efficacy and safety of topical becocalcidiol for the treatment of psoriasis vulgaris has been reported [39]. Becocalcidiol is a vitamin D analogue which did not cause hypercalcaemia or significant irritation in preclinical trials. In that study, the efficacy and safety of two dosing regimens of becocalcidiol ointment (low dose = 75 microg g(-1) once daily for 8 weeks; high dose = 75 microg g(-1) twice daily for 8 weeks) in the treatment of plaque-type psoriasis was analyzed. Outcomes included Physician's Static Global Assessment of Overall Lesion Severity (PGA) score; Psoriasis Symptom Severity (PSS) score; adverse events; and laboratory assessment. In that study high-dose becocalcidiol was statistically superior to vehicle [P = 0.002; 95% confidence interval (CI) 6.7-32.2], with 16 of 61 (26%) subjects achieving a PGA score of clear or almost clear. In all treatment arms, therapy was safe and well tolerated, with fewer subjects experiencing irritation than is reported in clinical studies using calcipotriol. The authors concluded that treatment with high-dose topical becocalcidiol for 8 weeks resulted in almost or complete clearing of moderate plaque-type psoriasis in over a quarter of patients and that the therapy was safe and well tolerated [39].

In 1996, a study demonstrated the efficacy and safety of oral 1,25(OH)2D3 in the treatment of psoriasis [40]. Of the 85 patients that received 1,25(OH)2D3 orally, 88.0% had after 36 month some improvement in their disease, 26,5%, 26,3%, and 25,3% had complete, moderate and slight improvement in their disease, respectively. Serum calcium concentrations and 24 h urinary calcium excretion increased, but were not outside the normal range. Bone mineral density of these patients was unchanged. A very important consideration for the use of orally administered 1,25(OH)2D3 is the dosing technique. To reduce unwanted effects on enhancing dietary calcium absorption, it is very important to provide 1,25(OH)2D3 at night time. Perez et al. [40] showed that as a result of this dosing technique, doses of 2 μg/ to 4 μg/night are well tolerated by psoriasis patients. Recently, the combination of acitretin and oral 1,25(OH)2D3 for successful therapy of plaque-type psoriasis has been reported [48].

Patients with psoriasis often need intermittent treatment for the whole of their lives. Vitamin D compounds have been shown not to result in tachyphylaxis during treatment of psoriatic lesions and can be continued indefinitely. They are effective and safe for the treatment of skin lesions that are often difficult to treat in psoriatic patients and that respond slowly. Additionally, vitamin D analogues are effective in the treatment of psoriasis in children and in HIV-patients.

Treatment of Scalp Psoriasis

It was shown that calcipotriol solution is effective in the topical treatment of scalp psoriasis [49]. 49 patients were treated twice daily over a four week period. 60% of patients on calcipotriol showed clearance or marked improvement vs. 17% in the placebo group. No side effects were reported.

Treatment of Nail Psoriasis

The occurrence of nail psoriasis has been reported in up to 50% of patients. Nails in general are very difficult to treat and respond slowly. Up to now, there has been no consistently effective treatment for psoriatic nails. Recently, it was shown that calcipotriol ointment is effective in the treatment of nail psoriasis [50].

Treatment of Face and Flexures

Although the use of calcipotriol ointment is not recommended on face and flexures due to irritancy, most patients tolerate vitamin D analogues on these sites. Recently, the tolerability and efficacy of calcitriol 3 microg g(-1) and tacrolimus 0.3 mg g(-1) ointment in chronic plaque psoriasis affecting facial and genitofemoral regions was analyzed [51]. In this double-blind, parallel, 6-week study, [50] patients were randomized in a 1 : 1 ratio to apply calcitriol or tacrolimus twice daily. The primary efficacy variable was the mean reduction of the target area score (TAS), and the secondary efficacy variable was the percentage of patients with the Physician's Global Assessment (PGA) score of 5 (clear) and 4 (almost clear) at the end of the study. Both calcitriol and tacrolimus were well tolerated. Although calcitriol induced perilesional erythema in a statistically significant higher proportion of patients than tacrolimus (55% vs. 16% at week 6; $P < 0.05$), it did not necessitate treatment discontinuation. At the end of the study, tacrolimus was significantly more effective than calcitriol based on a significant reduction of mean TAS (67% vs. 51%; $P < 0.05$) as well as more patients achieving complete or almost complete clearance by PGA (60% vs. 33%; $P < 0.05$). The authors concluded, that both calcitriol 3 microg g(-1) and tacrolimus 0.3 mg g(-1) are safe and well-tolerated therapeutic agents in the treatment of psoriasis in sensitive areas [51]. However, tacrolimus demonstrated a slightly more effective clinical outcome compared with calcitriol [51].

Treatment of Skin Lesions in Children

During the last years it has been shown that topical application of calcitriol ointment (3 μg of calcitriol per gram of petrolatum) is an effective, safe and reliable therapy to cure psoriatic skin lesions in children [52,53].

Treatment of Psoriatic Lesions in HIV-Patients

We have treated an HIV-positive patient suffering from psoriatic skin lesions with topical and oral calcitriol. The patient responded well and there was no evidence of enhancement in HIV-disease activity or alterations in the number of T-lymphocytes or CD4+ and CD8+ cells. Other case reports also demonstrate the efficacy and safety of vitamin D compounds in the treatment of psoriasis [54].

Combination of Vitamin D Compounds with other Therapies

It was shown that efficacy of topical treatment with vitamin D compounds in psoriasis can be increased by combination with other treatment regimens, including low dose oral cyclosporine (2 mg/ kg/ day), oral acitretin, topical dithranol, topical steroids, and UV-B or narrow band UV-B phototherapy [55-59]. Complete clearing or 90% improvement in PASI was reported in 50 % of patients treated with calcipotriol/cyclosporine vs. 11.8 % in the placebo/ cyclosporine arm. No difference was found in that study between the treatment arms in side effects.

Addition of calcipotriol ointment to oral application of acitretin (a vitamin A compound) was reported to produce a significantly better treatment response achieved with a lower cumulative dose of acitretin in patients with severe psoriasis, as compared with the group of patients treated with oral acitretin alone. The number of psoriasis patients reporting adverse events was similar between the two treatment arms [57].

Combined treatment with calcipotriol ointment (50 μg/g) and betametasone ointment was demonstrated to be slightly more effective and caused less skin irritation than calcipotriol used twice daily 58. As a consequence, calcipotriol is available in a combined formulation with betamethasone dipropionate. The efficacy and safety of the combined formulation of calcipotriol and betamethasone dipropionate when used over a 4-week period is well reported. Several publications discuss the safety of this product when used for 52 weeks, representing an option for maintenance therapy for psoriatic patients [60]. In an investigation using an economic model to simulate the costs and benefits [61], the cost-effectiveness of the two-compound formulation calcipotriol and betamethasone dipropionate was compared with other topical treatments commonly used in the therapy of moderately severe plaque psoriasis in Scotland. In that study, the two-compound formulation calcipotriol and betamethasone dipropionate were associated with reduced costs and superior outcomes as compared to other topical therapies.

Kragballe and coworkers reported that efficacy of topical calcipotriol treatment in psoriasis can be improved by combination with ultraviolet B (UVB) phototherapy. Combination therapy of psoriasis with topical calcipotriol and narrow-band UVB has also been shown to be very effective for the treatment of psoriatic plaques [59]. Experimental investigations demonstrated that calcipotriol is degraded by UV radiation, and suggested that calcipotriol should be applied after phototherapy but not immediately before. However, it was reported that the clinical effect of vitamin D analogues is not inactivated by subsequent UV exposure [62]. In that investigation, calcipotriol or maxacalcitol ointment was topically applied to psoriatic lesions of six patients immediately before or after phototherapy on the right or left side of the body, respectively. The topical application of vitamin D compounds either before or after irradiation by psoralen and UVA radiation (PUVA) or narrow-band UVB showed similar effects in all patients. The authors concluded that therapeutic effects of vitamin D compounds are not inactivated by subsequent irradiation with PUVA or UVB phototherapy.

Treatment of other Skin Disorders with Vitamin D Compounds

Earlier in the last century, vitamin D3 was used in dermatology in large pharmacological doses for the therapy of many skin diseases, including scleroderma, psoriasis, lupus vulgaris, and atopic dermatitis. However, these first attempts of vitamin D therapy in Dermatology were abandonned because of severe vitamin D intoxications that caused hypercalcemia, hypercalciuria, and kidney stones and because other new therapies were established for the treatment of these diseases.

Vitamin D Compounds and Ichthyosis

A clinical study showed the effectiveness of topical treatment with calcipotriol ointment on congenital ichthyoses [63]. Reduction in scaling and roughness on the calcipotriol-treated side was found in all patients with lamellar ichthyosis and bullous ichthyotic erythroderma of Brocq. The only patient with Comel-Netherton syndrome showed mild improvement, while the only patient suffering from ichthyosis bullosa of Siemens did not show any change in severity on the calcipotriol-treated as compared to the vehicle-treated lesions.

Vitamin D Compounds and Scleroderma

Case reports point at the efficacy of vitamin D compounds for the treatment of scleroderma. Humbert et al. [64] reported that oral administration of calcitriol improves skin involvement, probably via inhibition of fibroblast proliferation and dermal collagen deposition.

Vitamin D Compounds and Vitiligo

At present, many therapeutic agents are used for the treatment of vitiligo, but treatment remains a challenge. Investigations indicate that vitamin D analogues may be efficient and safe in the treatment of vitiligo. While some studies report about a successful therapy with topically applied vitamin D compounds including calcipotriol [65] or tacalcitol alone, others report about a successful therapy with topically applied vitamin D compounds in combination with UV- 66 or laser-therapy [67].

Vitamin D compounds and Skin Cancer

Many in vitro studies have shown strong antiproliferative and prodifferentiating effects of vitamin D compounds in VDR-expressing tumor cell lines, including malignant melanoma, squamous cell carcinoma and leukemic cells [18, 68]. In vivo studies supported these findings and demonstrated that active vitamin D compounds block proliferation and tumor progression of epithelial tumors in rats [69]. Moreover, it was demonstrated that administration of calcitriol reduced the number of lung metastases after implantation of lung carcinoma cells in mice [70]. Inhibition of growth of human malignant melanoma and colonic cancer xenografts was also shown in immune suppressed mice, but only a high doses of 1,25(OH)2D3 [71]. Not much is known regarding the effects of 1,25(OH)2D3 on neo-angiogenesis and on the formation of metastases in patients with malignant melanoma or squamous cell carcinoma of the skin.

Vitamin D Compounds and other Skin Diseases

Many case reports demonstrate positive effects of topical treatment with vitamin D compounds in a broad variety of skin diseases such as transient acantholytic dermatosis (Grovers disease), inflammatory linear verrucous epidermal naevus (ILVEN), disseminated superficial actinic porokeratosis, pityriasis rubra pilaris, epidermolytic palmoplantar keratoderma of Vorner, Sjögren-Larsson Syndrome, and others. These promising findings will have to be further evaluated in clinical trials.

Conclusion

Vitamin D compounds are effective and safe in the treatment of psoriasis. Moreover, they represent promising candidates that may be effective in the treatment of many other skin diseases.

References

[1] Holick MF, MacLaughlin JA, Clark MB, Holick SA, Potts JT, Anderson RR, Blank IH, Parrish JA, Elias P. Photosynthesis of previtamin D3 in human skin and the physiological consequences. *Science* 1980;210:203-5.

[2] Holick MF, MacLaughlin JA, Anderson RR, Parrish J. Photochemistry and photobiology of vitamin D. In: Regan JD, Parrish JA eds. *Photomedicine.* Plenum Press, New York. 1982:195-218.

[3] Holick MF, Smith E, Pincus S. Skin as the site of vitamin D synthesis and target tissue for 1,25-dihydroxyvitamin D3. *Arch Dermatol* 1987;123:1677-82.

[4] Holick MF. Photobiology, physiology and clinical applications for Vitamin D. In: Goldsmith LA, ed. *Physiology, biochemistry and molecular biology of the skin.* 2nd ed., Oxford University Press New York 1991:928-56.

[5] Bittiner B., Bleehen SS, Mac Neil S. 1α-25-(OH)2Vitamin D3 increases intracellular calcium in human keratinocytes. *Br J Dermatol* 1991; 124:12230-5.

[6] MacLaughlin JA, Cantley LC, Holick MF. 1,25(OH)2D3 increases calcium and phosphatidylinositol metabolism in differentiating cultured human keratinocytes. *J Nutr Biochem* 1990;1:81-7.

[7] Haussler MR. Vitamin D receptors: nature and function. *Annu Rev Nutr* 1986;6:527- 62.

[8] Haussler MR, Mangelsdorf DJ, Komm BS, Terpening CM, Yamaoka K, Allegretto EA, Baker AR, Shine J, McDonnell DP, Hughes M, Weigel NL, O'Malley BW. Molecular biology of the vitamin D hormone. *Recent Prog Horm Res* 1988;44:263- 305.

[9] Baker AR, Mc Donnell DP, Hughes M, Crisp TM, Mangelsdorf DJ, Haussler MR, Pike JW, Shine J, O'Malley BW. Cloning and expression

of full-length cDNA encoding human vitamin D receptor. *Proc Natl Acad Sci* USA 1988;85:3294-8.

[10] Yu VC, Deisert C, Andersen B, Holloway JM, Devary OV, Näär AM, Kim SY, Boutin JM, Glass CK, Rosenfeld MG. RXRβ: a coregulator that enhances binding of retinoic acid, thyroid hormone and vitamin D receptors to their cognate response elements. *Cell* 1991;67:1251-66.

[11] Leid M, Kastner P, Lyons R, Nakshatri H, Saunders M, Zacharewski T, Chen J, Staub A, Garnier J, Mader S, Chambon P. Purification, cloning, and RXR identity of the HeLa cell factor with which RAR or TR heterodimerizes to bind target sequences efficiently. *Cell* 1992;68:377-95.

[12] Milde P, Hauser U, Simon R, Mall G, Ernst V, Haussler MR, Frosch P, Rauterberg EW. Expression of 1,25-dihydroxyvitamin D3 receptors in normal and psoriatic skin. *J Invest Dermatol* 1991;97:230-9.

[13] Reichrath J, Münssinger T, Kerber A, Rochette-Egly C, Chambon P, Bahmer FA, Baum HP. In situ detection of retinoid-X receptor expression in normal and psoriatic human skin. *Br J Dermatol* 1995;133:168-75.

[14] Smith EL, Walworth NC, Holick MF. Effect of 1α-25-dihydroxyvitamin D3 on the morphologic and biochemical differentiation of cultured human epidermal keratinocytes grown under serum-free conditions. *J Invest Dermatol* 1986;86:709-14.

[15] Hosomi J, Hosoi J, Abe E, Suda T, Kuroki T. Regulation of terminal differentiation of cultured mouse epidermal cells by 1-alpha 25-dihydroxy-vitamin D3. *Endocrinol* 1983;113:1950-7.

[16] Gniadecki R, Serup J. Stimulation of epidermal proliferation in mice with 1 alpha, 25- dihydroxyvitamin D3 and receptor-active 20-EPI analogues of 1 alpha, 25- dihydroxyvitamin D3. *Biochem Pharmacol* 1995;49:621-4.

[17] Rigby WFC. The immunobiology of vitamin D. *Immunol today* 1988;9:54-8.

[18] Texereau M, Viac J. Vitamin D, immune system and skin. *Europ J Dermatol* 1992;2:258-64.

[19] Ranson M, Posen S, Mason RS. Human melanocytes as a target tissue for hormones: in vitro studies with 1α,25-dihydroxyvitamin D3, alpha-melanocyte stimulating hormone, and beta-estradiol. *J Invest Dermatol* 1988;91:593-8.

[20] Christophers E, Henseler T. Psoriasis of early and late onset: characterization of two types of psoriasis vulgaris. *J Am Acad Dermatol* 1985;13:450-6.

[21] Christophers E, Henseler T. Patient subgroups and the inflammatory pattern in psoriasis. *Acta Derm Venereol (Stockh)* 1989;69:88-92.

[22] Elder JT, Henseler T, Christophers E, Voorhees JJ, Nair RP. Of genes and antigens: the inheritance of psoriasis. *J Invest Dermatol* 1994;103:150S-3S

[23] Valdimarsson H, Baker BS, Jonsdittir I, Fry L. Psoriasis: a disease of abnormal keratinocyte proliferation induced by T lymphocytes. *Immunol Today* 1986;7:256-9.

[24] Lee RE, Gaspari AA, Lotze MT, Chang AE, Rosenberg SA. Interleukin 2 and psoriasis. *Arch Dermatol* 1988;124:1811-5.

[25] Barker JN, Jones ML, Mitra RS, Crockett Torab E, Fantone JC, Kunkel SL, Warren JS, Dixit VM, Nickoloff BJ. Modulation of keratinocyte derived interleukin-8 which is chemotactic for neutrophils and T lymphocytes. *Am J Pathol* 1991;139:869-76.

[26] Gottlieb AB. Immunologic mechanisms in psoriasis. *J Invest Dermatol* 1990;95:18S- 9S.

[27] Schlaak JF, Buslau M, Jochum W, Hermann E, Girndt M, Gallati H, Meyer zum Büschenfelde KH, Fleischer B. T cells involved in psoriasis vulgaris belong to the Th1 subset. *J Invest Dermatol* 1994,102:145-9.

[28] van Reijsen FC, Druijnzeel-Koomen CAFM, Kalthoff FS, Maggi E, Romagnani S, Westland JKT, Mudde GC. Skin-derived aeroallergen-specific T-cell clones of Th2 phenotype in patients with atopic dermatitis. *J Allergy Clin Immunol* 1992;90:184-92.

[29] Leung DY, Walsh P, Giorno R, Norris DA. A potential role for superantigens in the pathogenesis of psoriasis. *J Invest Dermatol* 1993;100:225-8.

[30] Zenz R, Eferl R, Kenner L, Florin L, Hummerich L, Mehic D, Scheuch H, Angel P, Tschachler E, Wagner EF. Psoriasis-like skin disease and arthritis caused by inducible epidermal deletion of Jun proteins. *Nature* 2005;437(7057):369-75.

[31] Chowaniec O, Jablonska S, Beutner EH, Proniewska M, Jarzabek Chorzelska M, Rzesa G. Earliest clinical and histological changes in psoriasis. *Dermatologica* 1981;163:42-51.

[32] MacLaughlin JA, Gange W, Taylor D, Smith E, Holick MF. Cultured psoriatic fibroblasts from involved and uninvolved sites have partial but

not absolute resistance to the proliferation-inhibition activity of 1,25-dihydroxyvitamin D3. *Proc Natl Acad Sci* USA 1985;82:5409-12.

[33] Morimoto S, Kumahara Y. A patient with psoriasis cured by 1α-hydroxyvitamin D3 *Med J Osaka Univ* 1985;35:3-4,51-4.

[34] Morimoto S, Yochikawa K, Kozuka T, Kitano Y, Imawaka S, Fukuo K, Koh E, Kumahara Y. An open study of vitamin D3 treatment in psoriasis vulgaris. *Br J Dermatol* 1986;115:421-9.

[35] Holick MF, Chen ML, Kong XF, Sanan DK. Clinical uses for calciotropic hormones 1,25-dihydroxyvitamin D3 and parathyroid hormone related peptide in dermatology: a new perspective. *J Invest Dermatol (Symp Proc)* 1996;1:1-9.

[36] Perez A, Chen TC, Turner A, Raab R, Bhawan J, Poche P, Holick MF. Efficacy and safety of topical calcitriol (1,25-dihydroxyvitamin D3) for the treatment of psoriasis. *Br J Dermatol* 1996;134:238-46.

[37] Kragballe K, Beck HI, Sogaard H. Improvement of psoriasis by topical vitamin D3 analogue (MC 903) in a double-blind study. *Br J Dermatol* 1988;119:223-30.

[38] van de Kerkhof PCM, van Bokhoven M, Zultak M, Czarnetzki BM. A double-blind study of topical 1α-25-dihydroxyvitamin D3 in psoriasis. *Br J Dermatol* 1989,120:661- 4.

[39] Helfrich YR, Kang S, Hamilton TA, Voorhees JJ. Topical becocalcidiol for the treatment of psoriasis vulgaris: a randomized, placebo-controlled, double-blind, multicentre study. *Br J Dermatol* 2007,157(2):369-74.

[40] Perez A, Raab R, Chen TC, Turner A, Holick MF. Safety and efficacy of oral calcitriol (1,25-dihydroxyvitamin D3) for the treatment of psoriasis. *Br J Dermatol* 1996;134:1070-8.

[41] Van de Kerkhof PC, Vissers WH. The topical treatment of psoriasis. *Skin Pharmacol Appl Skin Physiol* 2003;16:69-83.

[42] Kragballe K, Gjertsen BT, de Hoop D, Karlsmark T, van de Kerhof PCM, Larko O, Nieboer C, Roed-Petersen J, Strand A, Tikjob B. Double-blind right/left comparison of calcipotriol and betametasone valerate in treatment of psoriasis vulgaris. *Lancet* 1991;337:193-6.

[43] Tzaneva S, Hönigsmann H, Tanew A. Observer-blind, randomized, intrapatient comparison of a novel 1% coal tar preparation (Exorex R) and calcipotriol cream in the treatment of plaque type psoriasis. *Br J Dermatol* 2003;149:350-3.

[44] De Korte J, van der Valk PG, Sprangers MA, Damstra RJ, Kunkeler AC, Lijnen RL, Oranje AP, de Rie MA, de Waard-van der Spek FB, Hol CW, van de Kerkhof PC. A comparison of twice-daily calcipotriol

ointment with once-daily short-contact dithranol cream therapy: quality-of-life outcomes of a randomized controlled trial of supervised treatment of psoriasis in a day-care setting. *Br J Dermatol* 2008;158(2):375-81.

[45] Kragballe K, Barnes L, Hamberg KJ, Hutchinson P, Murphy F, Moller S et al. Calcipotriol cream with or without concurrent topical corticosteroid in psoriasis: Tolerability and efficacy. *Br J Dermatol* 1998;139:649-54.

[46] Zhu X, Wang B, Zhao G, Gu J, Chen Z, Briantais P, Andres P. An investigator-masked comparison of the efficacy and safety of twice daily applications of calcitriol 3 microg/g ointment vs. calcipotriol 50 microg/g ointment in subjects with mild to moderate chronic plaque-type psoriasis. *J Eur Acad Dermatol Venereol* 2007;21(4):466-472.

[47] Serup J. Calcipotriol irritation: Mechanism, diagnosis and clinical implication. *Acta Derm Venereol (Stockh) Abstract* 1994;186:42S.

[48] Ezquerra GM, Regana MS, Millet PU. Combination of acitretin and oral calcitriol for treatment of plaque-type psoriasis. *Acta Derm Venereol* 2007;87(5):449-50.

[49] Green C, Ganpule M, Harris D, Kavanagh G, Kennedy C, Mallett, R, Rustin M, Downes N. Comparative effects of calcipotriol (MC 903) solution and placebo (vehicle of MC 903) in the treatment of psoriasis of the scalp. *Br J Dermatol* 1994;130;483-7.

[50] Petrow W. Treatment of a nail psoriasis with calcipotriol. *Akt Dermatol* 1995;21:396- 400.

[51] Liao YH, Chiu HC, Tseng YS, Tsai TF. Comparison of cutaneous tolerance and efficacy of calcitriol 3 microg g(-1) ointment and tacrolimus 0.3 mg g(-1) ointment in chronic plaque psoriasis involving facial or genitofemoral areas: a double-blind, randomized controlled trial. *Br J Dermatol* 2007;157(5):1005-12.

[52] Saggese G, Federico G, Battini R. Topical application of 1,25 dihydroxyvitamin D3 (calcitriol) is an effective and reliable therapy to cure skin lesions in psoriatic children. *Eur J Pediatr* 1993;152:389-92.

[53] Perez A, Chen TC, Turner A, Holick MF. Pilot study of topical calcitriol (1,25-dihydroxyvitamin D3) for treating psoriasis in children. *Arch Dermatol* 1995;131:961-2.

[54] Gray JD, Bottomley W, Layton AM, Cotterill JA, Monteiro E. The use of calcipotriol in HIV-related psoriasis. *Clin Exp Dermatol* 1992;17(5):342-3.

[55] Grossman RM, Thivolet J, Claudy A, Souteyrand P, Guilhou JJ, Thomas P, Amblard P, Belaich S, de Belilovsky C, de la Brassinne M et al. A

novel therapeutic approach to psoriasis with combination calcipotriol ointment and very low-dose cyclosporine: a result of a multicenter placebo-controlled study. *J Am Acad Dermatol* 1994;31:68-74.

[56] Kerscher M, Volkenandt M, Plewig G, Lehmann P. Combination phototherapy of psoriasis with calcipotriol and narrow band UVB. *Lancet* 1993;342:923

[57] Cambazard, van de Kerkhof PCM, Hutchinson PE, and the Calcipotriol Study Group. Proceedings of the 3rd International Calcipotriol Symposium, *Munich Germany,* 23 March 1996.

[58] Ortonne JP. Calcipotriol in combination with betametasone diproprionate. Nouv. Dermatol 1994;13:736-751.

[59] Kragballe K. Combination of topical calcipotriol (MC 903) and UVB radiation for psoriasis vulgaris. *Dermatologica* 1990;181:211-4.

[60] Toole JW. Calcipotriol and betamethasone dipropionate for the treatment of psoriasis: a 52-week study. *Skin Therapy Lett* 2007;12 (4):1-3.

[61] Bottomley JM, Auland ME, Morais J, Boyd G, Douglas WS. Cost-effectiveness of the two-compound formulation calcipotriol and betamethasone dipropionate compared with commonly used topical treatments in the management of moderately severe plaque psoriasis in Scotland. *Curr Med Res Opin* 2007;23(8):1887-901.

[62] Adachi Y, Uchida N, Matsuo T, Horio T. Clinical effect of vitamin D3 analogues is not inactivated by subsequent UV exposure. *Photodermatol Photoimmunol Photomed 2008;*24(1):16-8.

[63] Lucker GP, van de Kerkhof PC, van Dijk MR, Steijlen PM. Effect of topical calcipotriol on congenital ichthyosis. *Br J Dermatol* 1994;131:546-50.

[64] Humbert P, Dupond JL, Agache P, Laurent R, Rochefort A, Drobacheff C, de Wazieres B, Aubin F. Treatment of scleroderma with oral 1,25-dihydroxyvitamin D3: evaluation of skin involvement using non-invasive techniques. Results of an open prospective trial. *Acta Derm Venereol (Stockh)* 1993;73:449-51.

[65] Kumaran MS, Kaur I, Kumar B. Effect of topical calcipotriol, betamethasone dipropionate and their combination in the treatment of localized vitiligo. *J Eur Acad Dermatol Venereol* 2006;20(3):269-73.

[66] Amano H, Abe M, Ishikawa O. First case report of topical tacalcitol for vitiligo repigmentation. *Pediatr Dermatol* 2008;25(2):262-4.

[67] Goldinger SM, Dummer R, Schmid P, Burg G, Seifert B, Läuchli S. Combination of 308-nm xenon chloride excimer laser and topical calcipotriol in vitiligo. *J Eur Acad Dermatol Venereol* 2007;21(4):504-8.

[68] Koeffler HP, Hirji K, Itri L. 1,25-dihydroxyvitamin D3: in vivo and in vitro effects on human preleukemic and leukemic cells. *Cancer Treat Rep* 1985;69:1399-407.

[69] Colston KW, Chander SK, Mackay AG, Coombes RC. Effects of synthetic vitamin D analogues on breast cancer cell proliferation in vivo and in vitro. *Biochem Pharmacol* 1992;44:693-702.

[70] Franceschi RT, Linson CJ, Peter CT, Romano PR. Regulation of cellular adhesion and fibronectin synthesis by 1α,25-dihydroxyvitamin D3. *J Biol Chem* 1987;262,4165-71.

[71] Eisman JA, Barkla DH, Tutton PJM. Suppression of in vivo growth of human cancer solid tumor xenografts by 1α,25-dihydroxyvitamin D3. *Cancer Res.* 1987;47:21-5.

Index

A

B

C

D

I

J

K

L

M

N

O

P

Q

R

S

T

U

V

W

X

Y

Z